AF693177

Table of Contents

1 Introduction

The intersection of pharmacology and forensic science has given rise to a critical field: pharmaceutical forensics. This discipline plays a vital role in understanding, mitigating, and preventing drug-related harm, ultimately contributing to patient safety. We delve into the intricacies of drug interactions and adverse reactions, providing a framework for healthcare professionals, legal experts, and researchers to navigate this complex landscape. This journey begins with understanding the fundamental principles that govern drug behavior in the body and how these principles can be applied to investigate and prevent medication-related incidents. By carefully examining the interplay between drugs and the human body, we can gain crucial insights into potential risks and develop strategies to safeguard patient well-being. The importance of this field is underscored by the increasing complexity of medication regimens and the potential for unforeseen consequences.

Forensic pharmacy, a cornerstone of this field, specifically addresses the investigation of drug-related incidents. These incidents can range from medication errors and adverse drug reactions to intentional drug misuse and product tampering. The forensic pharmacist's expertise lies in analyzing the circumstances surrounding these events, identifying the causative agents, and providing evidence-based conclusions. This meticulous approach involves gathering information from various sources, including patient medical histories, medication records, and laboratory analyses. The insights gained from these investigations contribute to improving medication safety practices and preventing future incidents. The forensic pharmacist acts as a detective, piecing together the puzzle of drug-related events to understand the underlying causes and contribute to a safer medication environment.

Drug interactions, a significant concern in modern healthcare, occur when the effects of one drug are altered by the presence of another drug, food, or other substance. These interactions can lead to either a reduction in the desired therapeutic effect or an increase in the risk of adverse reactions. Understanding the mechanisms of drug interactions is crucial for clinicians to make informed decisions regarding medication prescribing and patient monitoring. Several factors contribute to the likelihood of drug interactions, including the number of medications a patient is taking, the patient's age and overall health, and the specific properties of the drugs involved. Recognizing these factors is the first step in minimizing the potential for harm. For instance, a patient taking multiple medications for different conditions is at a higher risk of experiencing a drug interaction.

Adverse drug reactions (ADRs), another key focus of pharmaceutical forensics, are unintended and harmful responses to medications. These reactions can vary in severity from mild discomfort to life-threatening complications. ADRs can be classified into several categories, including predictable side effects related to the drug's known pharmacology, idiosyncratic reactions that are unpredictable and often immune-mediated, and dose-related toxicities that occur when drug levels exceed the therapeutic range. Recognizing and managing ADRs is critical to ensuring patient safety. This involves careful monitoring of patients for any signs or symptoms of adverse reactions, prompt intervention to mitigate harm, and reporting of suspected ADRs to regulatory authorities. This vigilant approach contributes to a broader understanding of drug safety profiles and informs future prescribing practices.

The consequences of overlooking drug interactions and ADRs can be profound, impacting both individual patients and the healthcare system as a whole. For patients, these events can lead to increased morbidity, prolonged hospital stays, and even mortality. From a healthcare perspective, the costs associated with managing drug-related complications place a significant burden on resources. Therefore, a proactive approach to preventing and managing these events is essential. This involves a multidisciplinary effort, including pharmacists, physicians, nurses, and other healthcare professionals working collaboratively to optimize medication therapy and minimize the risk of harm. Furthermore, empowering patients with the knowledge and tools to actively participate in their medication management is crucial. This includes educating patients about potential drug interactions and ADRs, encouraging them to report any unusual symptoms, and fostering open communication with their healthcare providers.

The complexity of human physiology, combined with the intricate pharmacology of medications, necessitates a rigorous and systematic approach to understanding and preventing drug-related harm. Pharmaceutical forensics provides the framework for this approach, integrating principles of pharmacology, toxicology, and forensic science to investigate and analyze drug-related incidents. By understanding the mechanisms of drug interactions and ADRs, we can develop effective strategies to mitigate risks and improve patient outcomes. This knowledge empowers healthcare professionals to make informed decisions about medication prescribing and patient monitoring, ultimately contributing to a safer and more effective medication use environment. The ongoing advancement of pharmaceutical forensics is critical for staying ahead of the evolving landscape of medications and ensuring the well-being of patients.

1.1 Forensic Pharmacy

Forensic pharmacy, a specialized field within pharmaceutical sciences, plays a crucial role in patient safety by applying forensic principles to medication-related incidents. It involves the investigation of drug-related events, including adverse drug reactions (ADRs), medication errors, and therapeutic drug monitoring, to identify the causative factors and prevent future occurrences. This detective-like approach combines knowledge of pharmacology, toxicology, and analytical chemistry to unravel the complex interplay of drugs within the human body. The goal is not simply to assign blame, but rather to understand the underlying mechanisms that contributed to the event and implement strategies to mitigate future risks. This systematic approach to analyzing medication-related incidents provides valuable insights for enhancing patient care and optimizing drug therapy.

The practice of forensic pharmacy often necessitates a detailed reconstruction of the patient's medication history. This involves meticulous examination of prescriptions, medication administration records, and patient interviews. Consider, for instance, a patient presenting with unexpected bleeding after starting a new anticoagulant. A forensic pharmacist might investigate the patient's concurrent use of other medications, including over-the-counter drugs and herbal supplements, to identify potential drug interactions that could have contributed to the bleeding. Dietary habits and lifestyle factors are also considered, as they can influence drug metabolism and efficacy. This comprehensive approach allows for a holistic understanding of the factors contributing to the adverse event, enabling targeted interventions to improve patient outcomes.

Beyond investigating individual cases, forensic pharmacy contributes to broader patient safety initiatives. By analyzing trends and patterns in medication-related incidents, forensic pharmacists can identify systemic issues within healthcare systems that contribute to medication errors or ADRs. For example, an analysis of reported ADRs might reveal a recurring problem with a particular drug formulation or a deficiency in medication reconciliation procedures during patient transitions. This information can then be used to implement targeted interventions, such as improved labeling, educational programs for healthcare professionals, or system-wide changes in medication management protocols. This proactive approach to identifying and addressing systemic issues is crucial for preventing future harm.

The analytical tools employed in forensic pharmacy are essential for understanding drug-related events. These tools, ranging from sophisticated chromatographic techniques to immunoassays, allow for the precise identification and quantification of drugs and their metabolites in biological samples. In cases of suspected drug overdose, for example, these analytical methods can confirm the presence and concentration of the suspected drug, providing crucial information for guiding treatment decisions. Furthermore, these techniques can help distinguish between an ADR caused by a drug itself and one caused by an underlying medical condition, aiding in accurate diagnosis and appropriate management. The ability to precisely measure drug levels also plays a critical role in therapeutic drug monitoring, ensuring that drug concentrations remain within the therapeutic range and minimizing the risk of toxicity.

Forensic pharmacy necessitates a strong understanding of drug interactions, which can significantly alter the effects of medications. Drug interactions occur when one drug influences the pharmacokinetics (absorption, distribution, metabolism, and excretion) or pharmacodynamics (mechanism of action) of another drug. A classic example is the interaction between warfarin, an anticoagulant, and certain antibiotics, which can enhance warfarin's anticoagulant effect, leading to an increased risk of bleeding. Forensic pharmacists play a critical role in identifying and evaluating potential drug interactions, educating healthcare professionals and patients about these risks, and recommending strategies to minimize adverse outcomes. This includes advising on appropriate dosage adjustments, alternative medications, or enhanced monitoring when potential interactions are unavoidable.

The field of forensic pharmacy is not limited to the investigation of adverse events; it also encompasses drug development and regulation. During the drug development process, forensic pharmacists contribute to the design and interpretation of clinical trials, evaluating the safety and efficacy of new medications. They also play a role in post-marketing surveillance, monitoring for rare or delayed ADRs that may not have been detected during clinical trials. This ongoing surveillance is crucial for ensuring the long-term safety of medications and informing updates to drug labeling and prescribing guidelines. The expertise of forensic pharmacists in analyzing complex drug-related data is invaluable for regulatory agencies in making informed decisions about drug approvals and safety warnings.

In the ever-evolving landscape of healthcare, the role of forensic pharmacy is becoming increasingly important. With the growing complexity of drug regimens and the increasing prevalence of polypharmacy, particularly in elderly populations, the potential for drug-related problems continues to rise. Forensic pharmacists are uniquely positioned to address these challenges, utilizing their expertise to prevent medication-related harm and improve patient outcomes. Their specialized knowledge in drug interactions, adverse drug reactions, and analytical techniques makes them essential members of the healthcare team, contributing significantly to the advancement of patient safety and the optimization of drug therapy. The continuous development of new medications and therapeutic approaches further underscores the need for forensic pharmacists to remain at the forefront of scientific advancements and adapt their skills to address the evolving challenges in medication safety.

1.2 Drug Interactions

The human body is a complex biochemical tapestry, and introducing drugs into this intricate system can sometimes lead to unexpected and even dangerous results. These results, known as drug interactions, occur when the effects of one drug are altered by the presence of another drug, food, supplement, or even a medical condition. Understanding these interactions is paramount for healthcare professionals and patients alike in ensuring safe and effective medication therapy. Drug interactions can manifest in a myriad of ways, from reducing the effectiveness of a medication to amplifying its side effects, or even creating entirely new adverse reactions.

One of the most common mechanisms of drug interactions is through the cytochrome P450 enzyme system in the liver. These enzymes are responsible for metabolizing many drugs, transforming them into forms that the body can more readily excrete. However, certain drugs can inhibit or induce these enzymes. For instance, if Drug A inhibits an enzyme that metabolizes Drug B, the levels of Drug B can rise in the bloodstream, potentially leading to toxicity.

Conversely, if Drug A induces an enzyme that metabolizes Drug B, it can accelerate the breakdown of Drug B, potentially rendering it ineffective. Grapefruit juice is a well-known example of a food that can inhibit certain cytochrome P450 enzymes, leading to increased blood levels of drugs like statins and some calcium channel blockers.

Beyond the liver's metabolic pathways, drug interactions can also occur at the site of absorption in the gastrointestinal tract. Some drugs require an acidic environment for optimal absorption. Taking antacids concurrently can reduce stomach acidity and hinder the absorption of these medications, diminishing their therapeutic effect. Similarly, drugs can interact within the bloodstream by competing for binding sites on plasma proteins. If Drug A displaces Drug B from these binding sites, it can increase the free, unbound concentration of Drug B, thereby increasing its activity and potential for side effects. This competition for protein binding can significantly influence the distribution of a drug throughout the body and its availability to reach its target site.

Drug interactions can also stem from pharmacodynamic mechanisms, where drugs influence each other's effects at the receptor level. This can involve synergistic effects, where the combined effect of two drugs is greater than the sum of their individual effects. For example, combining certain blood pressure medications can lead to a more substantial reduction in blood pressure than using either medication alone. Conversely, antagonistic effects can occur when two drugs oppose each other's actions. A classic example is the use of naloxone to reverse the effects of opioid overdose. Naloxone competes with opioids for binding sites at opioid receptors, effectively blocking the opioid's effects and restoring normal respiration.

The complexity of drug interactions underscores the importance of thorough medication reconciliation. This process involves reviewing a patient's complete medication list, including prescription drugs, over-the-counter medications, herbal supplements, and vitamins. Careful consideration of each medication's mechanism of action, potential interactions, and the patient's individual characteristics is crucial. Factors such as age, genetics, liver and kidney function, and underlying medical conditions can all influence a person's susceptibility to drug interactions. Open communication between patients and healthcare providers is vital. Patients should be encouraged to disclose all medications and supplements they are taking, including those obtained without a prescription. This comprehensive approach to medication management allows healthcare providers to identify potential drug interactions, adjust dosages as needed, and select alternative medications when necessary to minimize the risk of adverse events.

Furthermore, readily available resources, such as drug interaction databases and clinical decision support systems, provide valuable information to healthcare professionals. These tools can help identify potential drug interactions, assess their severity, and recommend appropriate management strategies. Ongoing monitoring of patients for signs and symptoms of drug interactions is equally important. Regular blood tests to measure drug levels, assessments of therapeutic response, and vigilance for any new or worsening side effects can help detect and manage drug interactions promptly. Education plays a pivotal role in empowering patients to actively participate in their medication safety. Patients should understand the importance of adhering to prescribed dosages and schedules, avoiding self-medication, and promptly reporting any unusual symptoms to their healthcare provider.

By integrating a thorough understanding of drug interaction mechanisms with comprehensive medication reconciliation, proactive monitoring, and patient education, we can significantly reduce the risk of adverse drug events and optimize medication therapy for improved patient outcomes. This proactive approach to patient care requires a collaborative effort among healthcare professionals, patients, and caregivers. Pharmacists, physicians, nurses, and other members of the healthcare team must work together to ensure that medication regimens are safe, effective, and tailored to each individual's needs. In the complex interplay of human physiology and pharmacology, vigilance and informed decision-making are paramount in safeguarding patient well-being.

1.3 Adverse Reactions

Adverse drug reactions (ADRs) represent a significant challenge in healthcare, impacting patient well-being and placing a substantial burden on healthcare systems. Understanding the intricacies of ADRs is paramount for all healthcare professionals involved in medication management. This chapter will delve into the multifaceted nature of ADRs, providing a framework for their classification, prediction, and effective management within the context of patient safety. We will explore the diverse spectrum of ADR manifestations, from common side effects to rare and potentially life-threatening reactions.

ADRs are broadly classified into several categories based on their underlying mechanisms and clinical presentation. Type A reactions, also known as augmented reactions, are predictable and dose-dependent, often representing an exaggeration of the drug's pharmacological effect. For instance, a patient taking a blood pressure medication might experience dizziness due to excessive lowering of blood pressure. Type B reactions, or bizarre reactions, are unpredictable and unrelated to the drug's known pharmacological action. These reactions are often idiosyncratic and can manifest as allergic reactions or other immunologically mediated responses. Type C reactions, or chronic reactions, arise from long-term drug exposure and may manifest as organ damage or other cumulative effects. Type D reactions, also referred to as delayed reactions, become apparent some time after drug exposure, often years later, and can include teratogenicity or carcinogenesis. Type E reactions, or end-of-use reactions, occur upon discontinuation of a drug and are characterized by withdrawal symptoms, highlighting the complexities involved in classifying and managing these diverse reactions.

Predicting ADRs is a crucial aspect of minimizing their occurrence. Several factors contribute to an individual's susceptibility to ADRs, including age, genetics, underlying health conditions, and concomitant medications. Pharmacogenomics plays an increasingly important role in identifying individuals with genetic variations that predispose them to specific ADRs. For example, variations in genes encoding drug-metabolizing enzymes can significantly influence drug clearance and subsequently increase the risk of adverse effects. Moreover, drug properties, such as lipophilicity and protein binding, can influence drug distribution and metabolism, further impacting the likelihood of ADRs. Polypharmacy, the concurrent use of multiple medications, significantly increases the risk of drug interactions and subsequent ADRs, emphasizing the importance of comprehensive medication reconciliation and careful consideration of potential drug interactions.

Managing ADRs requires a multifaceted approach. Prompt recognition and accurate diagnosis are essential for initiating appropriate interventions. In some cases, discontinuing the offending drug is sufficient to resolve the reaction. In other situations, symptomatic treatment may be necessary to alleviate the adverse effects. For severe reactions, such as anaphylaxis, immediate medical intervention is critical. Effective management also involves patient education about potential ADRs, emphasizing the importance of reporting any unusual symptoms to healthcare providers. This open communication empowers patients to actively participate in their own safety and contributes to a collaborative approach to medication management. Furthermore, understanding the temporal relationship between drug administration and the onset of symptoms is crucial for accurate diagnosis and appropriate management.

Reporting ADRs is a critical component of pharmacovigilance, the science of monitoring drug safety. Healthcare professionals play a vital role in reporting suspected ADRs to regulatory agencies, such as the Food and Drug Administration (FDA) in the United States or the European Medicines Agency (EMA) in Europe. These reports contribute to a collective understanding of drug safety profiles and inform regulatory decisions regarding drug labeling and usage recommendations. ADR databases serve as valuable resources for tracking and analyzing reported reactions, enabling the identification of emerging safety concerns and contributing to the continuous improvement of drug safety practices. These databases facilitate the detection of rare or delayed reactions that might not be apparent in clinical trials, further enhancing our understanding of long-term drug effects and enabling proactive measures to mitigate potential risks. By actively participating in ADR reporting, healthcare professionals contribute to a global effort to enhance patient safety and optimize medication use.

2 Drug Metabolism

The human body processes drugs through a complex series of chemical reactions, collectively known as drug metabolism. This intricate system transforms drugs into different chemical entities, generally making them more readily excretable from the body. Understanding this transformation is fundamental to pharmaceutical forensics, as it helps explain why individuals react differently to the same medication and how drug interactions can occur. This chapter will delve into the core principles of drug metabolism, highlighting the key pathways and enzymatic processes involved.

The liver is the primary organ responsible for drug metabolism, although other tissues, including the intestines, kidneys, and lungs, also play a role. Within the liver, a sophisticated network of enzymatic pathways orchestrates the modification of drugs. These pathways are broadly classified into Phase I and Phase II reactions. Phase I reactions, often involving oxidation, reduction, or hydrolysis, modify the drug's chemical structure, sometimes creating more reactive metabolites. Cytochrome P450 enzymes are central to Phase I metabolism, exhibiting remarkable versatility in their ability to catalyze the transformation of a wide range of drugs.

Phase II reactions involve the conjugation of the drug or its Phase I metabolites with endogenous molecules, such as glucuronic acid, sulfate, or glycine. This conjugation process generally increases the drug's water solubility, facilitating its excretion through the kidneys or bile. Several enzyme families, including UDP-glucuronosyltransferases, sulfotransferases, and glutathione S-transferases, are crucial for Phase II reactions. These distinct, yet interconnected, phases of metabolism work in concert to efficiently eliminate drugs from the system.

Enzyme kinetics plays a vital role in understanding the rate at which drugs are metabolized. The relationship between drug concentration and the rate of its metabolism is often described by the Michaelis-Menten equation, a fundamental concept in enzymology. This equation defines parameters like Vmax, the maximum rate of metabolism, and Km, the drug concentration at which metabolism proceeds at half its maximum rate. These parameters provide valuable insights into the efficiency of specific metabolic pathways and can predict how drug metabolism may be altered in different individuals or under different physiological conditions.

Genetic polymorphisms, variations in the DNA sequence of genes encoding drug-metabolizing enzymes, significantly influence individual responses to medications. These genetic differences can lead to altered enzyme activity, affecting the rate at which drugs are metabolized. Some individuals might possess gene variants that result in rapid metabolism, leading to lower drug concentrations and potentially reduced therapeutic efficacy. Conversely, slow metabolizers may experience higher drug concentrations, increasing the risk of adverse effects. Understanding these genetic variations is increasingly important in personalized medicine, allowing for tailored drug selection and dosing based on an individual's genetic profile.

Drug interactions often occur due to competition for the same metabolizing enzymes. When two drugs are metabolized by the same enzyme, they can compete for binding sites, potentially inhibiting the metabolism of one or both drugs. This inhibition can lead to elevated drug concentrations and an increased risk of adverse effects. Conversely, some drugs can induce the expression of specific metabolizing enzymes, increasing the rate of metabolism for other drugs. This induction can result in lower drug concentrations and reduced therapeutic efficacy.

Understanding the interplay between drug metabolism, enzyme kinetics, and genetic polymorphisms is paramount in pharmaceutical forensics. It allows for a deeper understanding of how drugs are processed by the body, explaining individual variability in drug response and predicting potential drug interactions. This knowledge is critical for investigating medication-related incidents, assessing the causality of adverse drug reactions, and ultimately, ensuring patient safety. Furthermore, appreciating the intricacies of drug metabolism highlights the importance of personalized medicine, where treatment strategies are tailored to each individual's unique metabolic profile. This approach promises to enhance drug efficacy and minimize the risk of adverse reactions, paving the way for safer and more effective drug therapies. The complexity of drug metabolism further emphasizes the need for continuous research and advanced analytical techniques to unravel the intricacies of drug behavior within the human body. This pursuit of knowledge is crucial for advancing pharmaceutical forensics and safeguarding patient well-being. Through sophisticated analytical methods, we can delve deeper into metabolic pathways and identify previously unknown metabolites, further enriching our understanding of drug disposition.

2.1 Metabolic Pathways

The human body processes drugs through a complex network of metabolic pathways, primarily occurring in the liver, but also in the intestines, kidneys, lungs, and even the skin. Understanding these pathways is fundamental to pharmaceutical forensics, as they directly influence drug efficacy, toxicity, and the potential for interactions. This intricate system can be broadly categorized into Phase I and Phase II reactions, each with distinct mechanisms and consequences.

Phase I reactions predominantly involve oxidation, reduction, and hydrolysis. These reactions often introduce or unmask a functional group on the drug molecule, making it more polar and therefore easier to excrete. A key player in Phase I metabolism is the cytochrome P450 (CYP) enzyme superfamily. These enzymes, particularly CYP3A4, CYP2D6, and CYP2C9, are responsible for metabolizing a vast majority of clinically used drugs. Variations in CYP enzyme activity, due to genetic polymorphisms or drug interactions, can significantly impact individual drug responses, leading to either therapeutic failure or toxicity. For instance, a patient with reduced CYP2D6 activity may experience increased drug levels and adverse effects when taking codeine, which relies on CYP2D6 for conversion to its active metabolite, morphine. Another example involves grapefruit juice, a known inhibitor of CYP3A4, which can elevate blood concentrations of drugs metabolized by this enzyme, such as statins and calcium channel blockers, increasing the risk of side effects.

Phase II reactions conjugate the drug or its Phase I metabolite with an endogenous molecule, like glucuronic acid, sulfate, or glutathione. This conjugation further increases the drug's water solubility and facilitates its elimination through urine or bile. Glucuronidation, the most common Phase II pathway, is catalyzed by uridine 5'-diphospho-glucuronosyltransferases (UGTs). Sulfation, another important pathway, utilizes sulfotransferases (SULTs) to attach a sulfate group to the drug. Glutathione conjugation, mediated by glutathione S-transferases (GSTs), is crucial for detoxifying reactive drug metabolites and preventing cellular damage. Genetic variations in these conjugating enzymes can also influence drug disposition and contribute to interindividual variability in drug response. For example, individuals with decreased UGT activity may experience increased levels of bilirubin, leading to jaundice, particularly when administered drugs that are glucuronidated. Similarly, variations in GST activity can affect an individual's susceptibility to drug-induced toxicity.

Beyond these two major phases, less common metabolic pathways exist, including acetylation and methylation. Acetylation, carried out by N-acetyltransferases (NATs), adds an acetyl group to the drug molecule. This pathway is particularly important for metabolizing certain antibiotics and anti-tuberculosis drugs. Methylation, catalyzed by methyltransferases, involves the transfer of a methyl group. While less prevalent in drug metabolism, it plays a role in the inactivation of certain neurotransmitters and hormones. Understanding these diverse pathways and their interplay is crucial for interpreting drug-related events in forensic investigations.

Investigating drug interactions necessitates a comprehensive understanding of the specific metabolic pathways involved. For example, a drug might inhibit or induce a specific CYP enzyme, affecting the metabolism of another drug that is a substrate for that same enzyme. This can lead to elevated drug levels and increased risk of toxicity, or conversely, reduced drug levels and therapeutic failure. Consider the interaction between ketoconazole, a potent CYP3A4 inhibitor, and simvastatin, a cholesterol-lowering drug metabolized by CYP3A4. Co-administration can lead to significantly elevated simvastatin levels, increasing the risk of rhabdomyolysis, a severe muscle tissue breakdown. Another example involves rifampin, a potent CYP3A4 inducer, which can accelerate the metabolism of warfarin, an anticoagulant. This interaction can reduce warfarin's effectiveness, potentially leading to thromboembolic events.

Further complicating the picture, drug metabolism can also be influenced by factors like age, gender, disease state, and diet. The elderly often have reduced liver function, leading to slower drug metabolism and increased susceptibility to drug accumulation and toxicity. Certain liver diseases, such as cirrhosis, can also impair drug metabolism. Dietary factors can either inhibit or induce enzyme activity, impacting drug disposition. Grapefruit juice, as mentioned earlier, is a classic example of a dietary inhibitor of CYP3A4. Conversely, cruciferous vegetables like broccoli can induce certain CYP enzymes. In forensic investigations, considering these factors is critical for accurate interpretation of drug concentrations and their potential contribution to adverse events.

The complexity of metabolic pathways underscores the importance of thorough investigation in pharmaceutical forensics. A complete understanding of these pathways allows for a more accurate assessment of drug interactions, adverse reactions, and ultimately, contributes to enhancing patient safety. By meticulously analyzing the interplay of various metabolic processes and individual patient factors, we can strive to minimize drug-related harm and optimize therapeutic outcomes.

2.2 Enzyme Kinetics

The interaction between a drug and its metabolizing enzyme can be understood through the lens of enzyme kinetics, a crucial aspect of pharmaceutical forensics. This field helps us predict how a drug will be processed within the body, and how this processing might be affected by other drugs or individual patient variability. The fundamental principles of enzyme kinetics provide a framework for understanding these complex processes. A key concept is the Michaelis-Menten equation, which describes the relationship between the rate of an enzyme-catalyzed reaction (v) and the concentration of the substrate (drug) [S]. This equation, v = (Vmax * [S]) / (Km + [S]), introduces two crucial parameters: Vmax and Km.

Vmax represents the maximum rate of the reaction when the enzyme is saturated with substrate. It effectively describes the enzyme's maximum capacity to process the drug. Imagine a factory worker with a limited number of hands; they can only assemble so many products per hour, even if there's an abundance of raw materials. Vmax is analogous to this maximum output. Km, on the other hand, is the substrate concentration at which the reaction velocity is half of Vmax. It reflects the enzyme's affinity for the substrate. A lower Km value indicates a higher affinity, meaning the enzyme binds and processes the drug efficiently even at low concentrations. Conversely, a higher Km signifies a weaker affinity, requiring higher drug concentrations for efficient metabolism.

Understanding these parameters is critical in predicting how different drugs might interact. For instance, consider two drugs metabolized by the same enzyme. If one drug has a significantly lower Km than the other, it will effectively outcompete the higher-Km drug for the enzyme's attention. This competition can lead to decreased metabolism of the higher-Km drug, potentially increasing its concentration in the body and raising the risk of adverse reactions. This competitive inhibition is a common mechanism of drug interactions, and understanding Km values helps predict these interactions.

Beyond competitive inhibition, enzyme kinetics also illuminates other types of drug interactions. Non-competitive inhibition, for example, occurs when a molecule binds to an enzyme at a site other than the active site, altering the enzyme's shape and reducing its activity. This type of inhibition affects Vmax without changing Km. Uncompetitive inhibition, another possibility, occurs when the inhibitor binds only to the enzyme-substrate complex. This affects both Vmax and Km, further complicating the drug's metabolic profile.

Furthermore, enzyme activity is not static. Various factors can influence enzyme function, impacting drug metabolism. Genetic variations, for instance, can lead to polymorphisms in drug-metabolizing enzymes, resulting in individuals who are "poor metabolizers," "intermediate metabolizers," "extensive metabolizers," or even "ultra-rapid metabolizers." These genetic differences can significantly alter drug response, requiring dose adjustments or even alternative therapies. For example, individuals with a genetic variant that results in reduced enzyme activity might experience increased drug exposure and a heightened risk of side effects. Conversely, ultra-rapid metabolizers might require higher doses to achieve therapeutic efficacy.

Disease states can also affect enzyme activity. Liver disease, for instance, can reduce the functional capacity of drug-metabolizing enzymes, impacting drug clearance. This reduced clearance can lead to drug accumulation and increased toxicity. Kidney disease can also affect drug elimination, though it doesn't directly impact enzyme kinetics. Understanding these influences is crucial for tailoring drug therapy to individual patients.

Drug interactions can further modulate enzyme activity. Enzyme induction, where one drug enhances the expression or activity of a metabolizing enzyme, can accelerate the metabolism of other drugs processed by the same enzyme. This can decrease their effectiveness, potentially leading to therapeutic failure. Enzyme inhibition, as discussed earlier, can have the opposite effect, reducing drug metabolism and potentially increasing the risk of adverse reactions. Finally, environmental factors such as diet and exposure to certain chemicals can influence enzyme activity. Grapefruit juice, for example, is a well-known inhibitor of the CYP3A4 enzyme, a major player in drug metabolism. Consuming grapefruit juice while taking certain medications can significantly increase drug levels, leading to adverse effects. Smoking, on the other hand, can induce certain enzymes, potentially decreasing the effectiveness of some drugs.

In conclusion, understanding enzyme kinetics is foundational in pharmaceutical forensics. By applying these principles, we can anticipate potential drug interactions, tailor therapies to individual patient variability, and ultimately contribute to safer and more effective drug use. From the Michaelis-Menten equation to the nuances of enzyme inhibition and induction, the principles discussed in this chapter equip healthcare professionals with the tools they need to navigate the complex world of drug metabolism. The interplay of these factors underscores the importance of considering individual patient characteristics, concomitant medications, and environmental influences when making therapeutic decisions.

3 Pharmacokinetic Principles

The human body acts as a complex terrain for drugs, with each medication navigating a unique journey from administration to elimination. This journey, governed by pharmacokinetic principles, dictates the drug's fate within the body, ultimately influencing its therapeutic effect and potential for adverse reactions. Understanding these principles is thus paramount in forensic pharmacy, enabling the investigation of drug-related incidents and contributing to improved patient safety. The core of pharmacokinetics lies in the interplay of absorption, distribution, metabolism, and excretion (ADME).

Absorption describes the process by which a drug enters the bloodstream from its site of administration. Factors influencing this process are multifaceted, encompassing the drug's physicochemical properties (like solubility and lipophilicity), the route of administration (oral, intravenous, topical, etc.), and the physiological state of the individual receiving the drug. For example, oral administration subjects a drug to the first-pass effect, where metabolism in the liver can significantly reduce the amount of drug reaching systemic circulation. Intravenous administration, bypassing the gastrointestinal tract, leads to rapid and complete absorption, making it crucial in emergency situations. Understanding these nuances is essential for interpreting drug levels and correlating them with observed effects.

Once absorbed, a drug embarks on its distribution throughout the body, reaching various tissues and organs. This process is influenced by factors such as blood flow, drug binding to plasma proteins, and the drug's ability to cross biological membranes like the blood-brain barrier. Highly perfused organs like the liver and kidneys receive a greater proportion of the drug initially, while tissues with limited blood supply, such as bone, experience slower drug distribution. Furthermore, the extent of protein binding can dramatically affect the free drug concentration, the fraction responsible for exerting pharmacological effects. A drug extensively bound to plasma proteins will have a smaller free fraction available to interact with its target, a critical consideration when evaluating drug interactions and potential toxicity.

Metabolism, primarily occurring in the liver, biotransforms drugs into metabolites, which may be more or less active than the parent compound. This process involves various enzymatic pathways, including cytochrome P450 enzymes, which can be subject to induction or inhibition by other drugs or environmental factors. Enzyme induction leads to accelerated drug metabolism, potentially reducing therapeutic efficacy, whereas enzyme inhibition can elevate drug levels, increasing the risk of adverse effects. Understanding these metabolic interactions is crucial for interpreting unexpected drug responses and potential toxicity. Genetic polymorphisms in drug-metabolizing enzymes also contribute to interindividual variability in drug response, further highlighting the complexity of predicting drug behavior in individual patients.

Excretion, the final stage of a drug's journey, involves the removal of the drug and its metabolites from the body. The kidneys play a dominant role in this process, filtering drugs from the bloodstream and eliminating them in the urine. Other routes of excretion include bile, feces, sweat, and exhaled air. Renal function significantly impacts drug clearance, and impaired kidney function can lead to drug accumulation and increased risk of toxicity. This necessitates dose adjustments for patients with renal impairment to avoid adverse events. Factors such as urine pH can also influence the rate of drug elimination, adding another layer of complexity to predicting drug behavior.

To quantify and predict drug behavior within the body, pharmacokinetic models are employed. These models, ranging from simple one-compartment models to more complex multi-compartment models, provide a mathematical framework for describing drug absorption, distribution, metabolism, and excretion. Parameters like volume of distribution, clearance, and half-life are derived from these models and provide valuable information for determining appropriate dosing regimens and predicting drug concentrations over time. Understanding these pharmacokinetic parameters is essential for interpreting drug levels in forensic investigations and establishing causality in drug-related incidents. Furthermore, these models help predict potential drug interactions by assessing the impact of one drug on the ADME of another. This predictive capacity is crucial for proactive risk management and personalized medicine, aiming to optimize drug therapy and minimize the risk of adverse events. In the context of forensic pharmacy, a thorough understanding of pharmacokinetic principles provides a foundation for investigating drug-related incidents. By considering the ADME processes and the factors that influence them, experts can reconstruct the timeline of drug exposure, assess the likelihood of a drug reaching toxic levels, and evaluate the contribution of drug interactions to observed adverse events. This knowledge contributes to a more accurate assessment of causality in medicolegal cases and aids in developing strategies for preventing future incidents.

3.1 Absorption & Distribution

The journey of a drug through the body is a complex odyssey governed by the principles of absorption and distribution. Understanding these principles is paramount in pharmaceutical forensics, as they dictate the drug's availability at its site of action and consequently, its efficacy and potential for adverse reactions. Absorption, the process by which a drug enters the bloodstream, is significantly influenced by the route of administration. Oral administration, the most common route, presents a series of challenges for a drug molecule. It must navigate the acidic environment of the stomach, withstand enzymatic degradation in the intestines, and permeate the intestinal lining to reach the portal circulation. Factors such as drug solubility, formulation, and gastrointestinal motility all play crucial roles in determining the extent and rate of absorption. Intravenous administration, on the other hand, bypasses these hurdles, delivering the drug directly into the systemic circulation, resulting in rapid and complete absorption. Other routes like intramuscular, subcutaneous, and transdermal administration offer varying degrees of absorption depending on factors such as blood flow to the site of administration and the drug's physicochemical properties.

Once absorbed, the drug embarks on the next leg of its journey: distribution. This process involves the reversible transfer of the drug from the bloodstream to the tissues and organs. The extent of distribution is influenced by several factors, including blood flow, capillary permeability, and the drug's affinity for plasma proteins and tissue components. Organs with high blood flow, such as the liver, kidneys, and heart, receive a greater proportion of the drug initially. However, the drug's ultimate distribution depends on its physicochemical properties, like lipid solubility and molecular size, which determine its ability to cross cell membranes and bind to tissue components. Highly lipophilic drugs can readily cross cell membranes and accumulate in fatty tissues, while hydrophilic drugs are largely confined to the extracellular fluid. Plasma protein binding also plays a significant role; drugs bound to plasma proteins, such as albumin, are effectively trapped within the bloodstream, limiting their distribution to tissues.

The interplay between blood flow and tissue affinity shapes the drug's concentration profile within the body. Consider a scenario where two drugs are administered simultaneously, one with a high affinity for muscle tissue and the other for adipose tissue. Despite similar initial distribution due to blood flow, over time, the muscle-seeking drug will accumulate preferentially in muscle, while the adipose-seeking drug will concentrate in fat. This differential distribution can have profound implications for both drug efficacy and toxicity. For instance, a drug that accumulates in adipose tissue may have a longer duration of action due to its slow release back into the circulation, potentially leading to prolonged exposure and increased risk of adverse effects.

Further complicating the picture is the existence of anatomical barriers that restrict drug access to certain compartments. The blood-brain barrier, a highly selective membrane protecting the central nervous system, presents a formidable challenge for drug delivery. Only drugs with specific physicochemical properties, such as high lipid solubility and low molecular weight, can effectively penetrate this barrier. This selective permeability has important implications for the treatment of neurological disorders, as drugs intended to act within the brain must be designed to overcome this barrier. Similarly, the placental barrier protects the developing fetus from potentially harmful substances, including many drugs. Understanding the factors that influence drug transfer across the placenta is crucial for ensuring the safety of both the mother and the fetus during pregnancy.

The distribution phase is not simply a passive process; it involves dynamic interactions between the drug and various physiological components. Drug transporters, specialized proteins embedded in cell membranes, play a critical role in facilitating or hindering drug movement across biological barriers. These transporters can actively pump drugs into or out of cells, influencing their distribution and elimination. For example, P-glycoprotein, a widely expressed efflux transporter, can limit drug absorption from the gut, enhance drug excretion from the kidneys, and restrict drug entry into the brain. Genetic variations in transporter expression can significantly impact individual drug responses, leading to interpatient variability in drug efficacy and toxicity.

Understanding the principles of absorption and distribution is fundamental to interpreting drug interactions and predicting adverse reactions. Alterations in these processes can have cascading effects on drug efficacy and safety. For example, a drug that inhibits intestinal P-glycoprotein can increase the absorption of another drug that is normally a substrate for this transporter, potentially leading to supratherapeutic drug levels and toxicity. Similarly, a drug that displaces another drug from plasma proteins can increase the free fraction of the displaced drug, leading to a higher concentration at the site of action and potentially enhancing its therapeutic or toxic effects. In forensic investigations, understanding these intricate relationships is crucial for establishing causality between drug exposure and observed adverse events. By meticulously analyzing the interplay between absorption, distribution, and other pharmacokinetic factors, we can unravel the complex puzzle of drug interactions and adverse reactions, ultimately contributing to safer and more effective drug therapy.

3.2 Metabolism & Excretion

The human body processes drugs through a complex interplay of absorption, distribution, metabolism, and excretion, often abbreviated as ADME. This chapter focuses on the latter two processes, metabolism and excretion, crucial stages that determine the duration and intensity of a drug's effect and ultimately its removal from the system. Understanding these processes is paramount in forensic pharmacy, particularly when investigating adverse drug reactions or drug-drug interactions. These concepts provide a framework for understanding how drugs are handled by the body and why certain individuals might be more susceptible to adverse effects.

Metabolism, primarily occurring in the liver, biotransforms drugs into metabolites. These metabolites can be pharmacologically active, inactive, or even toxic. The liver employs an array of enzymes, most notably the cytochrome P450 (CYP) superfamily, to catalyze these reactions. Different CYP enzymes exhibit varying substrate specificities, meaning they metabolize specific classes of drugs. This specificity is why genetic variations in CYP enzymes can significantly impact individual responses to medications. Some individuals, deemed "poor metabolizers," possess genetic variants that reduce enzyme activity, leading to slower drug metabolism and increased risk of adverse effects due to elevated drug levels. Conversely, "ultra-rapid metabolizers" possess genetic variants that increase enzyme activity, potentially leading to subtherapeutic drug levels and reduced efficacy. Considering these genetic variations is crucial in forensic investigations, especially when assessing causality in suspected ADRs.

The metabolic pathways involved can be broadly categorized as Phase I and Phase II reactions. Phase I reactions often involve oxidation, reduction, or hydrolysis, modifying the drug's chemical structure to create a more polar metabolite. This increased polarity facilitates excretion in the subsequent phase. Phase II reactions involve conjugation, where the drug or its Phase I metabolite is attached to an endogenous molecule, such as glucuronic acid, sulfate, or glycine. Conjugation further increases water solubility and promotes elimination. The specific metabolic pathway a drug follows depends on its chemical structure and the presence of specific enzymes. Understanding these pathways allows forensic pharmacists to predict potential drug interactions, as competition for the same metabolic enzymes can lead to altered drug levels and increased risk of toxicity.

Excretion, the process of removing drugs and their metabolites from the body, primarily occurs through the kidneys. Renal excretion involves glomerular filtration, tubular secretion, and reabsorption. Drugs and metabolites present in the bloodstream are filtered through the glomeruli into the renal tubules. Certain drugs are actively secreted into the tubules, while others may be passively reabsorbed back into the bloodstream. The balance of these processes determines the rate of drug elimination. Factors influencing renal function, such as age, disease, and concomitant medications, can significantly impact drug excretion and contribute to adverse drug reactions.

Beyond renal excretion, other routes of elimination exist, albeit usually playing a lesser role. Biliary excretion involves the transport of drugs and metabolites into the bile, which is then excreted into the intestines and ultimately eliminated in the feces. This pathway is particularly important for drugs with high molecular weights or those that are extensively conjugated. Pulmonary excretion, relevant for volatile substances like anesthetic gases, involves elimination through the lungs. Minor routes of excretion include sweat, saliva, and breast milk, which while quantitatively less significant, can still have forensic implications. For instance, the presence of drugs in breast milk can pose risks to nursing infants.

In forensic pharmacy, understanding the interplay between metabolism and excretion is essential for interpreting toxicological findings. For example, if a patient experiences an adverse reaction, analyzing drug and metabolite concentrations in biological samples can help determine if the reaction was caused by elevated drug levels due to impaired metabolism or excretion. Consider a scenario where a patient experiences excessive sedation after taking a standard dose of a benzodiazepine. If analysis reveals higher than expected plasma concentrations of the drug and lower levels of its metabolites, this could indicate impaired metabolism, potentially due to genetic factors or drug-drug interactions. Similarly, if a patient with impaired renal function experiences toxicity from a drug primarily excreted by the kidneys, this highlights the importance of considering renal function when prescribing medications.

Furthermore, understanding the pharmacokinetic properties of drugs, including their metabolism and excretion pathways, is essential in forensic investigations involving drug-related deaths.

By analyzing drug concentrations in postmortem samples and considering the individual's medical history and any potential contributing factors like co-ingested substances, forensic pharmacists can help determine the role of the drug in the cause of death.

In conclusion, the concepts of metabolism and excretion are foundational in pharmaceutical forensics. They provide a framework for understanding how drugs are handled by the body and how variations in these processes can lead to adverse drug reactions and drug-drug interactions. By applying this knowledge, forensic pharmacists can contribute to patient safety by helping to identify the causes of drug-related incidents and develop strategies to prevent them. The interplay between these processes, along with other pharmacokinetic factors, paints a complete picture of a drug's journey through the body, ultimately informing clinical decisions and contributing to safer medication practices.

3.3 Pharmacokinetic Models

Understanding drug behavior within the body is crucial for predicting and preventing adverse drug reactions and interactions. This relies heavily on pharmacokinetic models, which provide a mathematical framework for describing the absorption, distribution, metabolism, and excretion (ADME) of drugs. These models help us understand how drug concentrations change over time in different parts of the body, allowing us to optimize dosing regimens and minimize the risk of adverse events. We can use these models to explore various scenarios, such as different routes of administration or the impact of organ impairment.

Pharmacokinetic models are categorized based on their complexity and the assumptions they make about the body. Simpler models, like the one-compartment model, treat the body as a single, homogenous unit. This model assumes instantaneous drug distribution throughout the body and is useful for drugs that distribute rapidly. However, for drugs that exhibit complex distribution patterns, more sophisticated models are necessary. Two-compartment models, for instance, represent the body as two interconnected compartments: a central compartment representing highly perfused tissues like blood and organs, and a peripheral compartment representing tissues with slower drug distribution, such as muscle and fat. These models account for the different rates of drug distribution to various tissues, providing a more accurate representation of drug behavior. Even more complex models, such as multi-compartment models or physiologically-based pharmacokinetic (PBPK) models, incorporate physiological parameters like blood flow, tissue volumes, and drug-specific properties.

Parameters play a crucial role in defining the behavior of these models. Key parameters include volume of distribution (Vd), which relates the amount of drug in the body to its plasma concentration, indicating the extent of drug distribution into tissues. A larger Vd suggests greater drug distribution into tissues, while a smaller Vd indicates more drug remains in the plasma. Clearance (CL) represents the rate at which the drug is eliminated from the body. It combines information about metabolism and excretion and is crucial for determining drug dosage. Elimination half-life (t½) reflects the time it

takes for the drug concentration to decrease by half and is essential for understanding dosing frequency. Bioavailability (F) represents the fraction of the administered drug that reaches systemic circulation. It is particularly important when comparing different routes of administration, such as oral versus intravenous.

Applying these models in practical scenarios allows us to predict drug concentrations over time. For example, we can use these models to estimate the peak drug concentration (Cmax) and the time it takes to reach that peak (Tmax) after a single dose. This information is crucial for assessing the efficacy and safety of a drug. We can also use these models to determine the area under the concentration-time curve (AUC), which represents the total drug exposure over a given period. AUC is a useful parameter for comparing different formulations or dosing regimens.

In addition to predicting drug behavior in a 'typical' individual, pharmacokinetic models can also be individualized to account for patient-specific factors. Factors like age, weight, gender, genetics, and disease states can significantly impact drug ADME. By incorporating these factors into the models, we can tailor drug therapy to individual patients, optimizing treatment outcomes and minimizing the risk of adverse effects. For instance, patients with renal impairment may have reduced drug clearance, requiring dosage adjustments to avoid drug accumulation and toxicity. Similarly, genetic polymorphisms can affect enzyme activity, leading to altered drug metabolism and requiring personalized dosing strategies.

The application of pharmacokinetic models extends beyond individual patient care to encompass drug development and regulatory decision-making. In drug development, these models are used to guide the design of clinical trials, predict drug interactions, and select appropriate doses for different populations. Regulatory agencies use pharmacokinetic data to evaluate the safety and efficacy of new drugs and to make informed decisions about drug approvals.

Finally, advancements in computing power and modeling software have led to the development of more sophisticated and physiologically realistic pharmacokinetic models. These advanced models incorporate detailed physiological information and are capable of simulating drug behavior in specific organs and tissues. These models are increasingly used to investigate complex drug interactions, predict drug toxicity, and personalize drug therapy based on individual patient characteristics. They provide a powerful tool for improving our understanding of drug disposition and ultimately enhancing patient safety.

4 Drug Interactions Mechanisms

The human body processes drugs through a complex interplay of mechanisms, making it susceptible to interactions when multiple medications are introduced. These interactions can significantly alter a drug's intended therapeutic effect, leading to either a diminished response or an amplified, potentially toxic one. Understanding these intricate mechanisms is crucial for healthcare professionals to ensure patient safety and optimize treatment outcomes. We can broadly categorize drug interactions into two primary types: pharmacokinetic and pharmacodynamic.

Pharmacokinetic interactions occur when one drug affects the absorption, distribution, metabolism, or excretion (ADME) of another. Consider, for example, a drug that inhibits a specific enzyme responsible for metabolizing another medication. This inhibition can lead to elevated levels of the second drug in the bloodstream, potentially causing toxicity. Conversely, a drug that induces enzyme activity can accelerate the metabolism of another, reducing its effectiveness by decreasing its concentration below therapeutic levels. Absorption interactions can arise when drugs bind to each other in the gastrointestinal tract, hindering the absorption of one or both. Changes in gastric pH induced by one drug can also impact the solubility and absorption of others. Distribution interactions often involve competition for binding sites on plasma proteins. If one drug displaces another from these proteins, the unbound, free fraction of the displaced drug increases, potentially leading to heightened activity and possible toxicity. Finally, alterations in renal function caused by one drug can influence the excretion rate of another, further affecting its concentration and duration of action within the body.

Pharmacodynamic interactions, on the other hand, transpire at the drug's site of action, without necessarily impacting its concentration. These interactions can be synergistic, where the combined effect of two drugs is greater than the sum of their individual effects, or antagonistic, where the combined effect is less than the sum of their individual effects. Synergistic interactions can be beneficial in certain therapeutic contexts, such as combining antibiotics with different mechanisms of action to enhance bacterial killing. However, they can also lead to adverse effects if the potentiated effect is excessive. Antagonistic interactions can occur when two drugs compete for the same receptor site, diminishing the effect of one or both. This type of interaction can be exploited therapeutically, such as using naloxone to reverse opioid overdose. Alternatively, it can lead to treatment failure if the antagonism reduces the therapeutic effect of a necessary medication. Beyond receptor competition, pharmacodynamic interactions can involve complex downstream signaling pathways and physiological processes, making their prediction and management particularly challenging.

Understanding the specific mechanisms underlying a drug interaction is paramount for effective clinical management. For instance, if two drugs are known to interact through enzyme inhibition, adjusting the dosage of one or both drugs, or staggering their administration times, can mitigate the interaction's impact. Similarly, recognizing potential pharmacodynamic interactions allows clinicians to select alternative medications or closely monitor patients for adverse events. The interplay of multiple medications within a patient's regimen necessitates a comprehensive understanding of these intricacies.

Several factors contribute to the complexity of drug interactions. Polypharmacy, the concurrent use of multiple medications, significantly increases the risk of interactions. This is particularly relevant in elderly populations and patients with chronic conditions who often require numerous medications. Genetic polymorphisms in drug-metabolizing enzymes can also influence individual susceptibility to drug interactions. Patients with certain genetic variations may metabolize drugs more slowly or rapidly than others, altering their response to co-administered medications. Disease states, particularly those affecting liver or kidney function, can further complicate drug interactions by altering drug clearance and disposition. Finally, dietary factors and herbal supplements can also contribute to interactions, often through mechanisms involving enzyme modulation or competition for absorption or binding sites.

Understanding the intricacies of both pharmacokinetic and pharmacodynamic drug interactions requires careful consideration of all these factors. A thorough patient medication history, including prescription drugs, over-the-counter medications, and herbal supplements, is essential. Knowledge of a patient's genetic background, disease states, and dietary habits can further refine the assessment of potential interactions. Utilizing reliable drug interaction resources, such as databases and clinical decision support systems, can provide valuable information to clinicians. Ultimately, vigilance, careful monitoring, and proactive management are critical for preventing and mitigating the adverse consequences of drug interactions, ensuring patient safety and optimizing therapeutic outcomes. The subsequent chapters will delve deeper into specific examples of drug interactions and provide practical strategies for their management in various clinical scenarios. This foundational understanding of the underlying mechanisms provides a framework for navigating the complex landscape of drug interactions and promoting patient well-being.

4.1 Pharmacokinetic Interactions

The intricacies of pharmacokinetic interactions arise from the complex interplay between drugs as they navigate the body's systems for absorption, distribution, metabolism, and excretion. Understanding these interactions is crucial for preventing adverse drug reactions and ensuring therapeutic efficacy. These interactions can manifest in various ways, fundamentally altering the concentration of a drug at its site of action. This chapter will delve into the specific mechanisms by which these interactions occur, providing prac-

tical insights for healthcare professionals.
One prominent mechanism involves the alteration of drug absorption. A classic example is the interaction between antacids and certain antibiotics like tetracycline. Antacids, containing divalent cations such as calcium and magnesium, can chelate with tetracycline, forming insoluble complexes that reduce its absorption in the gastrointestinal tract. This leads to subtherapeutic antibiotic levels, potentially hindering the effectiveness of treatment and contributing to antibiotic resistance. Another example involves drugs affecting gastric pH, such as proton pump inhibitors, which can alter the solubility and thus the absorption of other medications dependent on specific pH ranges for optimal uptake.
Drug distribution, the process by which a drug reaches its target tissues, can also be significantly impacted by co-administered medications. Competition for plasma protein binding sites is a common mechanism. Many drugs bind reversibly to plasma proteins, such as albumin. When two drugs compete for the same binding site, the drug with lower affinity can be displaced, leading to an increase in its free, unbound fraction. This seemingly small change can have profound consequences, as the unbound fraction is pharmacologically active and can lead to increased drug effects, potentially reaching toxic levels. For example, the anticoagulant warfarin is highly protein-bound. Co-administration with a drug like sulfadiazine can displace warfarin, increasing the risk of bleeding.
Metabolic interactions, often involving the cytochrome P450 enzyme system in the liver, represent a significant source of pharmacokinetic variability. These enzymes play a vital role in drug

metabolism, and their activity can be induced or inhibited by other drugs. Enzyme induction, as seen with drugs like rifampin, can accelerate the metabolism of other drugs, leading to reduced therapeutic efficacy. Conversely, enzyme inhibition, a common interaction with drugs like ketoconazole, can decrease the metabolism of co-administered drugs, resulting in increased drug exposure and a higher risk of toxicity. Understanding the specific cytochrome P450 isoforms involved in a drug's metabolism is crucial for anticipating potential interactions.

Excretion, primarily via the kidneys, is the final stage of a drug's journey through the body, and it, too, can be influenced by drug interactions. Drugs can alter glomerular filtration rate, tubular secretion, or tubular reabsorption, affecting the elimination of other medications. For example, probenecid, typically used to treat gout, can inhibit the tubular secretion of penicillin, increasing penicillin's plasma concentration and prolonging its duration of action. This interaction can be beneficial in certain clinical scenarios, highlighting the potential for therapeutic exploitation of pharmacokinetic interactions. Conversely, some drugs can compete for the same renal transporters, leading to decreased clearance and potential toxicity.

The clinical implications of these pharmacokinetic interactions are far-reaching. They can range from minor alterations in drug efficacy to serious adverse events, including toxicity and even death. Therefore, recognizing potential interactions is crucial for ensuring patient safety. Factors such as age, genetics, and underlying disease states can further complicate the picture, underscoring the need for

personalized medicine approaches.
Effectively managing pharmacokinetic interactions requires a multifaceted approach. Thorough medication reconciliation, including over-the-counter drugs and herbal supplements, is essential. Understanding the pharmacokinetic properties of each medication, including its absorption, distribution, metabolism, and excretion pathways, is crucial for anticipating potential interactions. Utilizing drug interaction databases and consulting with pharmacists can provide valuable insights. Therapeutic drug monitoring, where feasible, can help optimize drug dosages and minimize the risk of adverse events.
In addition, patient education plays a critical role. Patients should be informed about the potential for drug interactions and instructed to report any unusual symptoms to their healthcare provider. Open communication between healthcare professionals and patients is paramount in managing these complex interactions and ensuring positive therapeutic outcomes. By integrating knowledge of pharmacokinetic principles with clinical practice, we can significantly enhance patient safety and optimize drug therapy. This proactive approach to managing drug interactions is a cornerstone of pharmaceutical forensics, ensuring the safe and effective use of medications.

4.2 Pharmacodynamic Interactions

Pharmacodynamic interactions represent a significant aspect of drug-related complications, often manifesting as unexpected or amplified therapeutic effects, or even adverse reactions. Unlike pharmacokinetic interactions, which alter drug absorption, distribution, metabolism, and excretion, pharmacodynamic interactions occur at the site of drug action. They involve complex interplay between drugs, impacting their effects on receptors, enzymes, or other physiological processes. Understanding these interactions is paramount for optimizing drug therapy and mitigating potential risks to patient safety.

One common mechanism of pharmacodynamic interaction is the additive or synergistic effect. This occurs when two drugs with similar pharmacological actions are administered concurrently, resulting in a combined effect greater than the sum of their individual effects. For example, combining two central nervous system depressants, such as an opioid analgesic and a benzodiazepine, can lead to profound sedation or even respiratory depression. Clinicians must carefully consider the potential for additive or synergistic effects when prescribing multiple medications with overlapping pharmacological properties. Dosage adjustments or alternative therapeutic strategies may be necessary to avoid potentially dangerous outcomes.

Another crucial mechanism is antagonistic interaction, where one drug opposes the action of another. This can arise from competition for the same receptor site or through different mechanisms impacting the same physiological pathway. For instance, the bronchodilator effect of beta-2 agonists, commonly used in asthma treatment, can be antagonized by beta-blockers prescribed for hypertension. This antagonism can lead to reduced bronchodilation and potential respiratory distress in susceptible individuals. Recognizing potential antagonistic interactions requires careful evaluation of patient medication lists and understanding the pharmacological properties of each drug.

Beyond additive and antagonistic effects, pharmacodynamic interactions can also manifest as alterations in drug response due to changes in receptor sensitivity or downstream signaling pathways. Chronic exposure to certain drugs can lead to receptor desensitization or tolerance, requiring higher doses to achieve the same therapeutic effect. Conversely, some drugs can potentiate the effects of others by enhancing receptor sensitivity or increasing the availability of downstream mediators. These complex interactions underscore the importance of individualized drug therapy and close monitoring of patient response.

The clinical implications of pharmacodynamic interactions can be profound, ranging from diminished therapeutic efficacy to life-threatening adverse reactions. For example, combining warfarin, an anticoagulant, with aspirin, an antiplatelet agent, can synergistically increase the risk of bleeding. Conversely, administering a nonsteroidal anti-inflammatory drug (NSAID) with an ACE inhibitor, commonly used for hypertension, can antagonize the antihypertensive effect and lead to uncontrolled blood pressure. These examples highlight the need for comprehensive medication reconciliation and careful consideration of potential pharmacodynamic interactions when prescribing new medications or managing existing drug regimens.

Understanding pharmacodynamic interactions is often complex

due to the multifaceted nature of drug actions and individual patient variability. Factors such as age, genetics, underlying disease states, and concomitant medications can all influence the likelihood and severity of pharmacodynamic interactions. Elderly patients, for instance, are often more susceptible to drug interactions due to age-related changes in drug metabolism and receptor sensitivity. Similarly, patients with hepatic or renal impairment may experience altered drug clearance, leading to increased drug exposure and a higher risk of adverse reactions.

To minimize the risk of pharmacodynamic interactions, healthcare professionals must employ a multi-pronged approach. Thorough medication reconciliation, including over-the-counter medications and herbal supplements, is essential. Educating patients about potential drug interactions and encouraging them to report any unusual symptoms is crucial for early detection and management of adverse reactions. Furthermore, utilizing drug interaction databases and consulting with pharmacists or clinical pharmacologists can provide valuable insights into potential drug interactions and help guide therapeutic decision-making.

Specific examples of pharmacodynamic interactions further illustrate their clinical relevance. Combining nitrates, used for angina, with phosphodiesterase-5 inhibitors, prescribed for erectile dysfunction, can lead to severe hypotension. This interaction occurs because both drugs increase intracellular cyclic guanosine monophosphate (cGMP), leading to excessive vasodilation. Another example is the interaction between monoamine oxidase inhibitors (MAOIs), used for depression, and tyramine-rich foods. MAOIs inhibit the breakdown of tyramine, which can lead to a hypertensive crisis if consumed in significant quantities.

Pharmacodynamic interactions are not always detrimental. In some cases, they can be exploited therapeutically. For example, combining certain antibiotics with a beta-lactamase inhibitor can enhance antibiotic efficacy by preventing bacterial resistance. Similarly, combining chemotherapy drugs with different mechanisms of action can improve cancer treatment outcomes by targeting multiple pathways involved in tumor growth. However, even in these instances, careful monitoring and dose adjustments are necessary to optimize therapeutic benefit and minimize the risk of adverse reactions.

5 Adverse Drug Reactions

Adverse drug reactions (ADRs) represent a significant challenge in healthcare, impacting patient well-being and placing a substantial burden on healthcare systems. Understanding the various facets of ADRs, from their classification and predictability to effective management and reporting, is paramount for all healthcare professionals. This chapter delves into the complexities of ADRs, equipping readers with the knowledge to navigate this critical aspect of patient care.

ADRs are broadly categorized into several types, each with distinct characteristics and clinical implications. Type A reactions, also known as augmented reactions, are predictable based on the drug's pharmacology. These reactions are often dose-dependent and represent an exaggeration of the drug's intended therapeutic effect, like excessive bleeding with anticoagulants. Type B reactions, on the other hand, are idiosyncratic and unpredictable, often involving immunological mechanisms or unusual individual sensitivities. These reactions can manifest as skin rashes, liver damage, or other unexpected effects, and are not related to the known pharmacology of the drug. Type C reactions are chronic reactions that arise from long-term drug exposure, such as tardive dyskinesia from prolonged antipsychotic use. Type D reactions are delayed reactions that may not become apparent until months or even years after drug exposure, a prime example being certain types of cancer related to past chemotherapy. Lastly, Type E reactions represent end-of-treatment effects, such as withdrawal symptoms experienced upon discontinuation of certain medications. Recognizing these distinct categories is crucial for accurate diagnosis and appropriate management.

Predicting ADRs involves a multifaceted approach, considering both patient-specific factors and drug properties. Patient demographics, such as age, gender, and genetic predisposition, play a significant role. Comorbidities and concomitant medications can further influence the risk of ADRs. Analyzing drug properties, including its chemical structure, metabolism, and potential for interaction with other drugs or food, is equally important. Specific laboratory tests, such as pharmacogenetic testing, can identify individuals at increased risk for certain ADRs based on their genetic makeup. Risk assessment tools, such as algorithms and scoring systems, are also available to help predict the likelihood of ADRs based on patient and drug characteristics.

Managing ADRs requires a prompt and systematic approach. The initial step involves identifying and confirming the suspected ADR, distinguishing it from other potential causes of the patient's symptoms. Once an ADR is suspected, de-challenge, or discontinuation of the suspected drug, is often the first course of action. In some cases, dose reduction may be sufficient. Supportive care measures, such as intravenous fluids or oxygen therapy, may be necessary to manage acute symptoms. Specific antidotes are available for certain drug-induced toxicities and should be administered promptly when indicated. Ongoing monitoring of the patient's condition is essential to assess the effectiveness of interventions and to detect any further complications.

Reporting suspected ADRs is a crucial component of pharmacovigilance, the science of monitoring drug safety. Healthcare professionals have a responsibility to report suspected ADRs to regulatory agencies, such as the Food and Drug Administration (FDA) in the United States or the Medicines and Healthcare products Regulatory Agency (MHRA) in the United Kingdom. These reports contribute to a broader understanding of drug safety profiles and can lead to updated warnings, label changes, or even drug withdrawals if necessary. Reporting mechanisms vary by country, but often involve online reporting systems or dedicated phone lines. Detailed information about the patient, the suspected drug, the observed reaction, and the outcome is typically required in these reports.

ADR databases play a crucial role in post-marketing surveillance and drug safety research. These databases compile reports of suspected ADRs from various sources, including healthcare professionals, patients, and pharmaceutical companies. Analyzing these data allows for the identification of potential safety signals, which are unexpected increases in the frequency or severity of ADRs. Databases like the World Health Organization's VigiBase and the FDA's Adverse Event Reporting System (FAERS) provide valuable resources for researchers and regulatory agencies to track and analyze ADR trends. These databases contribute significantly to our understanding of drug safety and inform decision-making related to drug approvals, warnings, and withdrawals. Through comprehensive data analysis, these repositories offer critical insights into the long-term safety profile of medications. They also serve as an essential tool for continuous monitoring and improvement of patient care.

5.1 Types of ADRs

Adverse drug reactions (ADRs) manifest in a variety of ways, each with unique characteristics and clinical implications. Understanding these different types is crucial for healthcare professionals to accurately diagnose, manage, and ultimately prevent patient harm. This chapter will delve into the classification of ADRs, providing a framework for recognizing their diverse presentations.

One primary distinction lies between predictable and unpredictable ADRs. Predictable reactions, often termed Type A reactions, stem from the known pharmacology of a drug. These are dose-dependent and account for the vast majority of ADRs encountered in clinical practice. For example, a common side effect of antihistamines is drowsiness, a direct consequence of their mechanism of action in the central nervous system. Managing such reactions often involves dose adjustment or switching to an alternative medication with a different pharmacological profile. Careful consideration of a drug's pharmacodynamic properties can often anticipate and mitigate these predictable effects.

Unpredictable reactions, or Type B reactions, are not directly related to the drug's known pharmacology. These reactions are often idiosyncratic, meaning they occur in a small percentage of patients and are not readily explained by the drug's typical effects. They are typically independent of dose and can range from mild skin rashes to severe, life-threatening conditions like Stevens-Johnson syndrome. Genetic predisposition, immunological factors, and underlying medical conditions can play a significant role in the development of these unpredictable reactions. Detecting and managing these reactions requires heightened vigilance and prompt discontinuation of the offending drug.

Further classifications within Type B reactions include immunologically mediated reactions, such as drug hypersensitivity reactions. These reactions involve the activation of the immune system, leading to allergic responses ranging from mild itching and hives to severe anaphylaxis. Understanding the underlying immunological mechanisms involved in these reactions is crucial for developing effective diagnostic and therapeutic strategies. Another subset includes idiosyncratic reactions, which remain largely unpredictable and often involve complex interactions between the drug, patient-specific factors, and environmental influences.

Metabolic idiosyncrasy represents another distinct category of ADRs. These reactions arise from individual variations in drug metabolism, often due to genetic polymorphisms affecting drug-metabolizing enzymes. These variations can lead to either increased or decreased drug clearance, resulting in altered drug exposure and potentially heightened risk of ADRs. For example, patients with certain genetic variations may metabolize a drug more slowly, leading to drug accumulation and an increased risk of toxicity. Pharmacogenomic testing can help identify patients at risk for these types of reactions, allowing for personalized drug selection and dosing.

Beyond these primary classifications, ADRs can also be categorized based on their time course. Acute reactions occur rapidly after drug administration, while delayed reactions may manifest days, weeks, or even months later. Chronic reactions develop over prolonged periods of drug exposure, often requiring careful monitoring and management to minimize long-term consequences. The time course of an ADR provides valuable clues in identifying the causative drug and understanding the underlying mechanisms involved.

Another crucial aspect of ADR classification considers the affected organ system. Hepatotoxicity, or drug-induced liver injury, is a serious ADR that can range from mild liver enzyme elevations to acute liver failure. Nephrotoxicity, affecting the kidneys, can manifest as impaired renal function or even acute kidney injury. Cardiotoxicity can encompass a range of cardiovascular complications, from arrhythmias to heart failure. Recognizing the specific organ system affected by an ADR is essential for targeted interventions and minimizing potential long-term damage.

Furthermore, understanding the severity of an ADR is critical for appropriate management. Mild reactions may only require symptomatic treatment or dose adjustment, while moderate reactions may necessitate hospitalization and specific therapeutic interventions. Severe reactions, including life-threatening conditions like anaphylaxis or Stevens-Johnson syndrome, require immediate medical attention and intensive care. Accurate assessment of ADR severity using standardized scales facilitates prompt and effective intervention. Finally, drug interactions can significantly contribute to the development and severity of ADRs. When multiple drugs are administered concurrently, they can interact with each other, leading to altered drug metabolism, increased drug concentrations, or enhanced pharmacological effects. These interactions can potentiate the risk of ADRs or create entirely new adverse events. Careful consideration of potential drug interactions is essential when prescribing multiple medications, especially in patients with complex medical conditions or those taking multiple medications. By recognizing the diverse types, mechanisms, and clinical presentations of ADRs, healthcare professionals can effectively monitor, manage, and ultimately prevent drug-related harm, promoting patient safety.

5.2 Predicting ADRs

Predicting adverse drug reactions (ADRs) is a critical aspect of patient safety and a cornerstone of responsible medication management. While it's impossible to foresee every potential ADR, a structured approach incorporating diverse data points can significantly enhance our ability to anticipate and mitigate risks. This chapter delves into the multifaceted landscape of ADR prediction, examining patient-specific factors, drug-specific properties, and the evolving tools available to healthcare professionals.

Consider a patient's genetic predispositions. Variations in genes coding for drug-metabolizing enzymes, like cytochrome P450s, can profoundly influence how individuals process medications. These genetic polymorphisms can lead to either accelerated or diminished metabolism, resulting in altered drug exposure and potentially increasing the risk of ADRs. Pharmacogenomic testing, while not routine for all medications, offers valuable insights, especially for drugs with a narrow therapeutic index or known susceptibility to genetic variations in metabolism.

Beyond genetics, a patient's age significantly impacts drug response. Infants, with their immature organ systems, and older adults, often experiencing age-related decline in organ function, are particularly vulnerable to ADRs. Physiological changes associated with aging, such as reduced renal clearance and altered drug distribution, necessitate dosage adjustments and heightened vigilance for potential adverse events. Concomitant diseases further complicate the picture. Liver and kidney disease, for instance, can impair drug clearance, increasing the risk of drug accumulation and toxicity. Heart failure can alter drug distribution, while conditions like diabetes can influence drug metabolism and increase susceptibility to certain ADRs.

Drug properties themselves offer valuable clues for predicting ADRs. The chemical structure of a drug, its lipophilicity, and its protein-binding characteristics can influence its distribution and elimination, impacting the likelihood of ADRs. For example, highly lipophilic drugs may accumulate in adipose tissue, leading to prolonged exposure and increased risk of toxicity. Drugs with high protein binding compete for binding sites, potentially displacing other medications and altering their free concentrations, thereby increasing the risk of ADRs. Furthermore, the drug's pharmacological mechanism of action can provide insights into potential adverse effects. Drugs that act on multiple receptor subtypes, for example, are more likely to exhibit a broader range of adverse effects compared to drugs with more selective actions.

Dose-response relationships are fundamental to understanding ADRs. Higher doses generally increase the risk of both on-target and off-target adverse effects. Furthermore, the route of administration can influence the onset and severity of ADRs. Intravenous administration, for example, delivers the drug directly into the systemic circulation, resulting in rapid onset of action and potentially increasing the risk of acute reactions. Conversely, oral administration allows for gradual absorption, often mitigating the intensity of initial effects but potentially leading to delayed onset ADRs related to cumulative exposure.

The duration of therapy also plays a role in ADR prediction. Long-term use of certain medications, such as corticosteroids, can lead to a cumulative increase in the risk of specific ADRs like osteoporosis or adrenal suppression. Therefore, the benefit-risk assessment should be continuously reevaluated during long-term therapy, and strategies for minimizing long-term risks should be implemented.

Polypharmacy, the concurrent use of multiple medications, exponentially increases the risk of drug interactions and ADRs. Each additional medication adds to the complexity of drug interactions, potentially altering the pharmacokinetics and pharmacodynamics of other drugs and increasing the likelihood of adverse events.

Emerging technologies are revolutionizing ADR prediction. Data mining and machine learning algorithms are being employed to analyze vast datasets of patient information, including electronic health records, genomic data, and drug exposure information, to identify patterns and predict individual patient susceptibility to ADRs. These in silico approaches hold immense promise for personalized medicine and proactive risk mitigation. Furthermore, the development of in vitro models using human cells and tissues allows for preclinical screening of drug candidates for potential ADRs, providing valuable information before clinical trials.

Finally, consider drug-drug interactions. Certain drug combinations can synergistically or antagonistically interact, altering their respective pharmacokinetic profiles or pharmacodynamic effects. For example, one drug might inhibit the metabolism of another, leading to increased drug exposure and a higher risk of ADRs. Conversely, two drugs might compete for the same receptor, diminishing their therapeutic effects and potentially leading to adverse events. Understanding these complex interactions is crucial for predicting and mitigating potential ADRs in patients receiving multiple medications. Resources like drug interaction databases and clinical decision support systems can provide valuable information to healthcare professionals when prescribing medications for patients on complex drug regimens.

5.3 Managing ADRs

Effective management of adverse drug reactions (ADRs) is paramount for patient safety and positive therapeutic outcomes. This involves a multi-pronged approach encompassing prompt recognition, assessment, and appropriate intervention strategies. Recognizing an ADR requires vigilance and a thorough understanding of the patient's medication history, underlying medical conditions, and presenting symptoms. It's crucial to differentiate ADRs from disease progression or other co-existing conditions. Careful evaluation of temporal relationships between drug administration and symptom onset is essential, along with considering the pharmacological properties of the suspected drug. Often, a detailed patient interview is the most valuable tool in uncovering potential ADRs.

Assessment of the suspected ADR involves determining its severity and causality. Severity is graded based on standardized scales, ranging from mild discomfort to life-threatening reactions. Causality assessment employs established algorithms like the Naranjo Algorithm or the World Health Organization-Uppsala Monitoring Centre (WHO-UMC) system. These algorithms consider factors such as temporal relationship, dechallenge (improvement upon drug discontinuation), rechallenge (recurrence of symptoms upon re-administration), and alternative explanations for the observed symptoms. Accurate causality assessment helps guide decisions regarding future drug therapy.

Managing ADRs requires a tailored approach based on the specific reaction and its severity. Mild reactions, such as nausea or rash, may only require symptomatic treatment or dosage adjustments. Moderate reactions might necessitate temporary discontinuation of the offending drug, while severe reactions, like anaphylaxis or Stevens-Johnson syndrome, demand immediate cessation of the drug and aggressive supportive care. In some instances, specific antidotes or pharmacological interventions may be necessary to counteract the ADR. For example, administering epinephrine in anaphylactic reactions or corticosteroids in severe hypersensitivity reactions can be life-saving.

Beyond immediate management, preventing future ADRs is equally crucial. This involves thorough medication reconciliation, ensuring that patients are not prescribed medications with known interactions or contraindications based on their individual risk factors. Patient education plays a vital role; empowering patients with knowledge about potential ADRs, their symptoms, and when to seek medical attention can significantly improve outcomes. Encouraging patients to maintain an updated list of their medications, including over-the-counter drugs and supplements, is essential for preventing unintended interactions and subsequent ADRs.

Pharmacists are uniquely positioned to contribute to ADR management. Their expertise in drug interactions, pharmacodynamics, and pharmacokinetics enables them to proactively identify potential ADR risks and provide tailored recommendations to both patients and healthcare providers. Pharmacists can educate patients about proper medication administration, potential side effects, and the importance of adherence to prescribed regimens. They can also work collaboratively with physicians to optimize drug therapy, minimizing the risk of ADRs while maximizing therapeutic benefits.

Utilizing available resources, such as drug information databases and clinical decision support systems, further enhances ADR management. These resources provide up-to-date information on drug interactions, adverse effects, and recommended monitoring parameters. Regularly consulting these resources allows healthcare professionals to stay informed about emerging drug safety concerns and make informed decisions regarding patient care. Moreover, participating in ongoing professional development activities related to ADR management and pharmaco vigilance strengthens clinical expertise and promotes best practices.

Documentation of ADRs is crucial for both individual patient care and broader public health initiatives. Accurate and complete documentation in the patient's medical record facilitates communication among healthcare providers, enabling consistent management strategies. Furthermore, reporting ADRs to national and international pharmacovigilance centers contributes to the ongoing surveillance of drug safety. These reports contribute to a collective body of knowledge that can lead to updated drug labeling, regulatory action, and improved prescribing practices.

Integrating pharmacogenomic information into ADR management holds immense promise for personalized medicine. Genetic variations can influence drug metabolism and disposition, predisposing individuals to certain ADRs. By identifying patients with specific genetic markers, healthcare providers can tailor drug selection and dosage to minimize the risk of ADRs and optimize therapeutic efficacy. As pharmacogenomic testing becomes more readily available, its integration into clinical practice will play an increasingly important role in preventing and managing ADRs.

5.4 Reporting ADRs

Effective reporting of Adverse Drug Reactions (ADRs) forms the cornerstone of pharmacovigilance, playing a crucial role in safeguarding public health. It provides invaluable data that continuously refines our understanding of drug safety profiles, ultimately leading to safer medication practices for everyone. This chapter will delve into the intricacies of ADR reporting, empowering you with the knowledge and skills necessary to contribute meaningfully to this vital process. We will explore the "who, what, when, where, and how" of ADR reporting. Understanding these core elements is paramount for effective communication and ultimately, improved patient safety.

Identifying an ADR is the first, and often most challenging, step in the reporting process. Not all adverse events experienced by a patient taking a medication are necessarily ADRs. A thorough assessment, considering the patient's medical history, concomitant medications, and the temporal relationship between drug administration and the onset of the adverse event, is essential. Differentiating between symptoms caused by the underlying disease and those potentially attributable to the medication requires careful clinical judgment. Sometimes, seemingly minor events can be indicative of a serious underlying ADR, emphasizing the importance of meticulous observation and documentation. Look for unusual symptoms, those not typically associated with the patient's condition, or an unexpected exacerbation of pre-existing conditions.

Once a suspected ADR is identified, the next step involves gathering comprehensive information about the event. This includes details about the patient, such as age, gender, and relevant medical history. Document the specific medication involved, including the dose, route of administration, and duration of therapy. Crucially, provide a detailed description of the adverse event itself. Precisely characterize the nature of the reaction, its severity, the time of onset, and its duration. If the reaction subsided upon discontinuation of the drug or with a change in dosage, note this as well. This detailed information forms the backbone of a thorough ADR report.

The timing of ADR reporting varies depending on the severity of the reaction and local regulations. Serious ADRs, defined as those resulting in death, hospitalization, disability, or a life-threatening event, necessitate immediate reporting. For less severe reactions, reporting timelines may be more flexible, but prompt reporting is always encouraged. Delays can hinder the timely identification of potential drug safety issues, potentially exposing more patients to unnecessary risk. Familiarize yourself with the specific reporting guidelines and timelines established by your institution and relevant regulatory authorities.

Knowing where to report a suspected ADR is critical for ensuring that the information reaches the appropriate channels. In many countries, national pharmacovigilance centers or regulatory agencies are responsible for collecting and analyzing ADR reports. Healthcare professionals often have designated internal reporting procedures within their institutions. Pharmaceutical companies also play a crucial role in monitoring the safety of their products and have established systems for receiving ADR reports. Understanding the appropriate reporting pathways within your specific context is essential.

Reporting methods for ADRs vary, but the goal remains consistent: to provide clear, concise, and accurate information. Many regulatory agencies and institutions provide standardized reporting forms that facilitate this process. These forms typically prompt for the key information outlined earlier, ensuring a comprehensive report. Online reporting systems are increasingly common, streamlining the submission process and allowing for efficient data collection. Regardless of the specific method used, accurate and detailed documentation is paramount.

Consider a scenario where a patient receiving a newly approved antibiotic develops a severe skin rash. The healthcare provider, recognizing the potential for a serious ADR, immediately documents the reaction. They meticulously record the characteristics of the rash, its onset relative to the initiation of the antibiotic, and any other associated symptoms. This information is then reported promptly to the national pharmacovigilance center using the designated online reporting system. This timely and detailed report contributes to the ongoing surveillance of the antibiotic's safety profile. The accumulated data from multiple reports can reveal patterns and potential safety signals, ultimately leading to informed decisions regarding the drug's continued use.

In another instance, a pharmacist notices an unusual clustering of similar adverse events among patients receiving a specific medication. Recognizing the potential significance of this observation, the pharmacist initiates an investigation. They gather detailed information about the affected patients, including their medical histories, concomitant medications, and the specific adverse events experienced. This information is compiled into a comprehensive report and submitted to the pharmaceutical company that manufactures the medication. This proactive approach facilitates the early detection of potential safety concerns, potentially preventing further harm.

Reporting ADRs is not merely a regulatory requirement; it's a professional responsibility and a crucial contribution to patient safety. Every report adds another piece to the complex puzzle of drug safety. By diligently observing, documenting, and reporting suspected ADRs, we collectively contribute to a safer medication environment for all.

5.5 ADR Databases

The bedrock of effective pharmacovigilance rests upon the robust collection, analysis, and dissemination of information regarding adverse drug reactions. This is where Adverse Drug Reaction (ADR) databases become indispensable tools. These repositories serve as centralized hubs for accumulating reports of suspected ADRs from various sources, including healthcare professionals, patients, and pharmaceutical companies. They provide crucial data for identifying potential safety signals, understanding the incidence and prevalence of ADRs, and ultimately, enhancing patient safety by informing clinical decision-making and regulatory actions. These databases vary in scope, from national systems like the FDA's Adverse Event Reporting System (FAERS) in the United States and the Yellow Card Scheme in the UK, to international initiatives such as the World Health Organization's VigiBase. Each database possesses its own unique characteristics in terms of reporting requirements, data collection methods, and accessibility.

Understanding the nuances of these different databases is essential for anyone involved in pharmacovigilance. For instance, some databases, like FAERS, are publicly accessible, allowing researchers and the public to scrutinize reported adverse events. Others maintain restricted access, limiting data sharing to authorized parties due to privacy concerns and proprietary information. Navigating these differences requires careful consideration of the specific research question, data requirements, and ethical considerations. It is also critical to be aware of the limitations inherent in spontaneous reporting systems, as these databases rely on voluntary submissions and may not capture the true incidence of ADRs due to underreporting.

Despite their limitations, ADR databases offer invaluable insights into the safety profiles of medications. They play a pivotal role in signal detection, the process of identifying potential associations between a drug and an adverse event. This process involves analyzing large datasets for statistically significant increases in the reporting of specific ADRs associated with a particular drug. Signal detection can trigger further investigations, such as epidemiological studies or clinical trials, to confirm or refute the suspected association. The information gleaned from these analyses can lead to updates in drug labeling, including warnings about potential risks, or even the withdrawal of a drug from the market if the risks outweigh the benefits.

Beyond signal detection, ADR databases contribute significantly to understanding the broader landscape of drug safety. By analyzing aggregated data, researchers can identify risk factors for specific ADRs, such as age, gender, concomitant medications, and underlying medical conditions. This information can be used to develop risk stratification tools and personalize treatment strategies to minimize the likelihood of adverse events. Furthermore, ADR databases enable researchers to track the long-term safety of medications, providing insights into rare or delayed-onset reactions that may not be apparent in pre-marketing clinical trials.

Effective utilization of ADR databases requires a thorough understanding of data mining techniques and statistical analysis. Researchers need to be proficient in querying databases, filtering data based on specific criteria, and applying statistical methods to identify meaningful patterns and trends. This often involves complex data manipulation and interpretation, necessitating specialized training and expertise. Furthermore, understanding the specific data elements collected within each database is essential for accurate data analysis. For instance, knowing how different databases classify and code adverse events is crucial for comparing data across different systems.

The increasing volume and complexity of data within ADR databases has spurred the development of sophisticated data analysis tools. These tools utilize advanced algorithms and machine learning techniques to automate data processing, identify hidden patterns, and predict potential drug safety issues. While these tools hold great promise for enhancing pharmacovigilance, their effective application requires careful validation and interpretation of the results. Human oversight remains crucial to ensure the accuracy and reliability of the analyses.

In the context of pharmaceutical forensics, ADR databases serve as an essential resource for investigating suspected drug-related harm. They provide valuable information about the known safety profile of a drug, which can be used to assess the plausibility of a causal relationship between a drug and an observed adverse event. Furthermore, access to detailed case reports within these databases can provide insights into the clinical presentation, time course, and management of specific ADRs, aiding in the forensic investigation.

Moving forward, the continued development and refinement of ADR databases will be crucial for advancing patient safety. This includes improving data quality, enhancing data sharing and interoperability between different systems, and developing more sophisticated analytical tools. Collaboration between regulatory agencies, pharmaceutical companies, healthcare professionals, and patients is essential to maximize the potential of these databases to prevent drug-related harm and ensure the safe and effective use of medications. The future of pharmacovigilance hinges on the robust utilization of these invaluable resources.

6 Forensic Techniques

The cornerstone of any forensic investigation, particularly within the pharmaceutical realm, lies in the meticulous application of analytical methods. These methods serve as the investigative lens, allowing us to peer into the complex interplay of drugs and the human body. Consider, for instance, the scenario of a patient presenting with unexpected symptoms after initiating a new medication. The analytical toolkit at our disposal becomes crucial for unraveling the potential connection between the medication and the adverse event. This might involve identifying the drug and its metabolites in biological fluids like blood or urine, quantifying their concentrations to assess exposure levels, and even examining tissue samples for evidence of drug-induced damage.

The selection of an appropriate analytical method hinges on several factors, including the nature of the drug in question, the matrix being analyzed (e.g., blood, urine, tissue), the sensitivity required, and the availability of resources. Chromatographic techniques, coupled with mass spectrometry (MS), are frequently employed due to their high sensitivity and specificity. Gas chromatography-mass spectrometry (GC-MS) is well-suited for volatile compounds, while liquid chromatography-mass spectrometry (LC-MS) is preferred for analyzing non-volatile and thermally labile compounds. Immunoassays, leveraging the specificity of antibody-antigen interactions, offer a rapid and cost-effective approach for screening purposes, although they may lack the sensitivity of chromatographic methods. In some instances, more specialized techniques like capillary electrophoresis or nuclear magnetic resonance spectroscopy may be necessary.

Beyond the identification and quantification of drugs and their metabolites, forensic techniques also encompass the assessment of drug purity and the detection of adulterants or contaminants. This is particularly relevant in cases of suspected counterfeit medications or drug tampering. Sophisticated analytical techniques, such as high-performance liquid chromatography (HPLC) with diode-array detection or inductively coupled plasma mass spectrometry (ICP-MS), can be employed to pinpoint the presence of impurities or unexpected components. Imagine a scenario involving a batch of medications suspected of being contaminated with heavy metals. ICP-MS would be an invaluable tool for confirming the presence and concentration of such contaminants, providing crucial evidence for regulatory action.

The data generated by these analytical methods represent just one piece of the puzzle. The true power of forensic techniques lies in the skillful interpretation of these data to establish causality and reconstruct the sequence of events leading to an adverse reaction or drug interaction. This requires a deep understanding of pharmacokinetic and pharmacodynamic principles, coupled with meticulous attention to detail. Consider the case of a patient experiencing an unexpected bleeding event after starting a new anticoagulant medication. Analyzing the patient's blood for the drug concentration alone is insufficient. The forensic expert must also consider factors such as the patient's age, renal function, concomitant medications, and genetic predisposition to bleeding to determine whether the observed drug concentration is within the therapeutic range or if it contributed to the bleeding event.

Interpreting analytical data often involves comparing the measured drug concentrations with established therapeutic ranges. However, these ranges are not absolute and must be considered in the context of individual patient variability. Furthermore, the presence of drug metabolites can significantly impact the observed effects. Some metabolites may possess pharmacological activity of their own, while others may be inactive or even toxic. A thorough understanding of the metabolic pathways of a drug is essential for accurately interpreting the analytical findings.

Case studies serve as invaluable teaching tools in pharmaceutical forensics, illustrating the practical application of analytical methods and data interpretation. Consider the case of a patient presenting with severe liver toxicity after taking a combination of herbal supplements. Analyzing the supplements revealed the presence of a previously unknown contaminant, a hepatotoxic alkaloid. This finding not only helped to explain the patient's symptoms but also led to a product recall, preventing further harm to others. Such case studies highlight the critical role of forensic techniques in safeguarding public health. They demonstrate how the meticulous application of scientific principles, combined with careful data interpretation, can unravel complex drug-related events and contribute to safer medication practices. These real-world examples bring the abstract concepts of pharmaceutical forensics to life, showcasing their tangible impact on patient care and emphasizing the importance of rigorous investigation in unraveling the enigma of drug interactions and adverse reactions. Through this detailed analysis, we gain valuable insights into the practical application of forensic techniques, ultimately contributing to the broader goal of enhancing patient safety and preventing future medication-related harm.

6.1 Analytical Methods

The cornerstone of pharmaceutical forensics lies in the ability to accurately identify and quantify drugs and their metabolites in various biological matrices. This chapter explores the analytical methods employed in this critical process, providing a foundation for understanding how these techniques contribute to unraveling the complexities of drug interactions and adverse reactions. We will delve into the intricacies of these methodologies, highlighting their strengths and limitations in different forensic contexts.

Chromatographic techniques, particularly gas chromatography (GC) and high-performance liquid chromatography (HPLC), are central to pharmaceutical forensic analysis. GC, coupled with mass spectrometry (GC-MS), offers exceptional sensitivity and specificity for volatile compounds. Its ability to separate complex mixtures and provide definitive identification makes it invaluable in analyzing drugs with diverse chemical structures. HPLC, coupled with various detectors like UV-Vis, fluorescence, and mass spectrometry (LC-MS), extends analytical capabilities to non-volatile and thermally labile compounds. The versatility of HPLC makes it suitable for a wide range of pharmaceuticals, including peptides, proteins, and other macromolecules.

Immunoassays provide rapid, high-throughput screening for specific drugs or drug classes. Techniques like enzyme-linked immunosorbent assays (ELISA) and radioimmunoassays (RIA) leverage the specificity of antibody-antigen interactions to detect and quantify target analytes in biological samples. While highly sensitive, immunoassays can be susceptible to cross-reactivity with structurally similar compounds, potentially leading to false positives. Consequently, confirmatory testing using more specific methods, such as GC-MS or LC-MS, is often necessary.

Spectroscopic techniques, including UV-Vis, infrared (IR), and nuclear magnetic resonance (NMR) spectroscopy, play crucial roles in drug identification and structural elucidation. UV-Vis spectroscopy, while less specific than other methods, offers a rapid and simple approach for initial drug screening and quantitation. IR spectroscopy provides valuable information about the functional groups present in a molecule, aiding in compound identification. NMR spectroscopy, with its ability to provide detailed structural information, is essential for characterizing unknown compounds and confirming the identity of suspected drugs.

The selection of the appropriate analytical method depends on several factors, including the nature of the drug being analyzed, the matrix in which it is present, the sensitivity and specificity required, and the available resources. For instance, analyzing volatile drugs in blood may necessitate GC-MS, while analyzing non-volatile drugs in urine might favor LC-MS. In cases where rapid screening is paramount, immunoassays can be employed, followed by confirmatory analysis using more definitive techniques.

Sample preparation is a critical step in the analytical process, ensuring the analyte is extracted and purified from the complex biological matrix. Techniques like liquid-liquid extraction, solid-phase extraction, and protein precipitation are commonly employed to isolate the drug of interest while removing interfering substances. Proper sample preparation minimizes matrix effects, enhances analytical sensitivity, and improves the accuracy and reliability of results.

Data interpretation in pharmaceutical forensics requires careful consideration of various factors, including the analytical method employed, the limitations of the technique, and the potential for interferences. Establishing a chain of custody for samples is crucial to maintain the integrity of the evidence and ensure its admissibility in legal proceedings. Quality control measures, including the use of certified reference materials and regular instrument calibration, are essential for producing reliable and defensible data.

The interpretation of analytical results must consider the pharmacokinetic and pharmacodynamic properties of the drug in question. Understanding the drug's absorption, distribution, metabolism, and excretion profile is crucial for interpreting drug concentrations in biological samples. Factors such as the time elapsed since drug administration, the route of administration, and individual patient variability can significantly influence drug levels.

Furthermore, interpreting analytical data requires considering the potential for drug interactions and their impact on observed drug concentrations. For instance, one drug may inhibit the metabolism of another, leading to elevated levels of the parent drug and potentially increased risk of adverse reactions. Conversely, one drug may induce the metabolism of another, resulting in lower drug levels and potentially reduced therapeutic efficacy.

In cases involving adverse drug reactions, analytical methods can help establish a causal link between the drug and the observed adverse event. By quantifying drug levels and identifying potential metabolites, forensic scientists can assess whether the drug was present at a concentration sufficient to cause the observed effects. This information can be crucial in determining the cause of an adverse reaction and in developing strategies to prevent future occurrences.

Finally, the integration of analytical data with other clinical information, such as patient medical history, concomitant medications, and symptoms, is essential for a comprehensive understanding of the case. A holistic approach, combining analytical findings with clinical context, allows for a more accurate assessment of drug-related incidents and facilitates informed decision-making in patient care.

6.2 Data Interpretation

The crux of pharmaceutical forensics lies in the ability to interpret complex data derived from analytical techniques. This involves more than simply reading numbers; it requires a deep understanding of the underlying scientific principles and the ability to draw meaningful conclusions that can inform clinical decisions and improve patient safety. This process begins with a thorough understanding of the specific analytical method employed, its limitations, and potential sources of error. Whether it's chromatography, mass spectrometry, or immunoassays, a strong grasp of the technique's intricacies is paramount for accurate interpretation.

Consider, for instance, a case involving a suspected drug overdose. Analysis of blood samples might reveal the presence of multiple drugs and their metabolites. Interpreting this data requires understanding the pharmacokinetic properties of each drug, including its absorption rate, distribution volume, metabolism, and elimination pathway. Furthermore, the interaction between these drugs must be considered, as one drug can alter the metabolism or elimination of another, leading to unexpected concentrations. This intricate interplay of factors requires a meticulous approach to data analysis, considering all variables to arrive at a valid conclusion.

Beyond individual drug properties, patient-specific factors also play a crucial role in data interpretation. A patient's age, weight, gender, genetics, and underlying health conditions can all influence drug disposition and response. For example, a patient with impaired liver function might metabolize a drug more slowly, leading to higher blood concentrations and an increased risk of adverse effects. This information must be integrated into the data analysis process to accurately assess the contribution of drug levels to the observed clinical picture.

Moreover, interpreting data in the context of an adverse drug reaction requires careful consideration of the temporal relationship between drug administration and the onset of symptoms. The time course of drug concentrations, coupled with the patient's clinical presentation, can provide crucial clues about the likelihood of a causal relationship. For instance, a rapid onset of symptoms shortly after drug administration might suggest an immediate hypersensitivity reaction, while a delayed onset could indicate a more complex immunological or metabolic mechanism.

The interpretation of analytical data is not a solitary endeavor. It often involves collaboration with other healthcare professionals, including clinicians, pharmacists, and toxicologists. This interdisciplinary approach is essential for integrating diverse perspectives and expertise to arrive at the most accurate and comprehensive interpretation. Sharing data and interpretations across disciplines facilitates a holistic understanding of the case, leading to more informed decisions regarding patient care.

Furthermore, the interpretation process benefits from a structured approach, involving a systematic review of all available data, including patient history, medication records, laboratory results, and analytical findings. This comprehensive evaluation ensures that all relevant information is considered, minimizing the risk of overlooking crucial details that could impact the interpretation. A structured approach also promotes transparency and reproducibility, enabling other experts to review the data and interpretations and arrive at similar conclusions.

In addition to the scientific principles, ethical considerations must also guide the interpretation of data. Objectivity and impartiality are paramount. Interpretations should be based solely on the available evidence, without bias or preconceived notions. This commitment to ethical practice ensures that the interpretations are reliable and trustworthy, contributing to the integrity of the forensic investigation and the pursuit of patient safety.

Finally, staying abreast of the latest scientific advancements and regulatory guidelines is essential for ensuring accurate and up-to-date data interpretation. The field of pharmaceutical forensics is constantly evolving, with new analytical methods and technologies emerging regularly. Continuing education and professional development are crucial for staying informed about these advancements and incorporating them into practice. This ongoing learning process allows practitioners to refine their interpretive skills and contribute to the advancement of the field. By adhering to these principles, practitioners can effectively utilize data interpretation to unravel the complexities of drug interactions and adverse reactions, ultimately contributing to improved patient safety.

6.3 Case Studies

A seemingly straightforward case involved a 72-year-old woman admitted for acute exacerbation of congestive heart failure. Her medication regimen included digoxin for heart rate control and warfarin for atrial fibrillation. Upon admission, her international normalized ratio (INR), a measure of blood clotting time, was significantly elevated, indicating a heightened risk of bleeding. A thorough medication review revealed she had recently started taking St. John's Wort, an herbal supplement often used for mild to moderate depression. St. John's Wort is a known inducer of the cytochrome P450 enzyme CYP3A4, which metabolizes warfarin. This interaction resulted in increased warfarin metabolism, leading to higher than intended INR levels and the subsequent bleeding risk. This case highlights the importance of obtaining a complete medication history, including over-the-counter medications and herbal supplements, to identify potential drug interactions. Educating patients about the risks of combining prescription medications with herbal remedies is crucial for preventing such complications.

In a more complex scenario, a 45-year-old man presented with severe muscle weakness and pain. He was diagnosed with rhabdomyolysis, a condition involving muscle breakdown. He was taking simvastatin for high cholesterol and erythromycin for a bacterial infection. Erythromycin is a known inhibitor of CYP3A4, the primary enzyme responsible for simvastatin metabolism. This inhibition led to a significant increase in simvastatin concentrations, exceeding the therapeutic range and causing muscle toxicity. This case underscores the critical role of understanding drug metabolism pathways and the potential for drug interactions when multiple medications are prescribed concurrently. Clinicians must be vigilant in recognizing the potential for drug interactions, particularly when prescribing medications metabolized by the same enzyme system.

A perplexing case involved a 60-year-old woman who experienced sudden cardiac arrest. She had a history of hypertension and was taking metoprolol, a beta-blocker. Post-mortem analysis revealed significantly elevated metoprolol levels in her blood. Further investigation unveiled she had been taking grapefruit juice daily. Grapefruit juice inhibits CYP3A4, the enzyme responsible for metoprolol metabolism. This inhibition resulted in a substantial increase in metoprolol levels, contributing to the fatal cardiac event. This case emphasizes the importance of patient education regarding food-drug interactions. Even seemingly innocuous substances like grapefruit juice can have profound effects on drug metabolism and lead to serious adverse events.

Another case involved an 80-year-old man who developed acute kidney injury following initiation of an ACE inhibitor for hypertension. He was concurrently taking nonsteroidal anti-inflammatory drugs (NSAIDs) for arthritis. NSAIDs can reduce renal blood flow, while ACE inhibitors can also impact kidney function. The combined effect of these two drugs led to a significant decline in kidney function, resulting in acute kidney injury. This case demonstrates the importance of considering pharmacodynamic interactions, where the combined effects of drugs on the same physiological system can lead to adverse outcomes.

A challenging case involved a 35-year-old woman with epilepsy who experienced breakthrough seizures despite taking her prescribed anticonvulsant medication, phenytoin. Investigation revealed she had recently started taking a combined oral contraceptive pill.

Some oral contraceptives can increase the metabolism of phenytoin through enzyme induction. This interaction led to subtherapeutic phenytoin levels, resulting in a loss of seizure control. This case highlights the complexity of drug interactions and the need for careful consideration of individual patient factors and medication regimens.

A final illustrative case involves a 55-year-old man admitted to the hospital with severe gastrointestinal bleeding. He had a history of peptic ulcer disease and was taking warfarin for atrial fibrillation. He had recently been prescribed a course of ibuprofen for back pain. NSAIDs like ibuprofen can irritate the gastrointestinal lining and increase the risk of bleeding, especially in patients also taking anticoagulants like warfarin. This combination of drugs synergistically increased the risk of gastrointestinal bleeding, resulting in a life-threatening event. This case emphasizes the importance of evaluating the combined risks of medications, especially when prescribing drugs with overlapping adverse effect profiles. A careful risk-benefit assessment is essential for ensuring patient safety.

These case studies serve as potent reminders of the intricate interplay between drugs within the human body. Each scenario underscores the critical need for a thorough understanding of drug interactions, metabolism, and individual patient factors. By integrating this knowledge into clinical practice, healthcare professionals can effectively mitigate risks, optimize therapeutic outcomes, and ultimately enhance patient safety.

7 Patient Safety Strategies

Effective patient safety related to medication requires a multi-faceted approach, blending proactive risk assessment with continuous monitoring and responsive interventions. Consider the complexity of the human body – its intricate network of systems, each influencing the other. A seemingly innocuous medication can trigger a cascade of unforeseen consequences, particularly when interacting with other drugs or pre-existing conditions. This inherent complexity demands a vigilant approach to medication management, one that anticipates and mitigates potential risks before they escalate into adverse events.

Risk assessment forms the cornerstone of patient safety strategies. Think of it as a preemptive strike against potential harm. By identifying patients at heightened risk of adverse drug reactions or interactions, healthcare professionals can tailor medication regimens accordingly. This requires a thorough understanding of patient-specific factors, including age, comorbidities, genetic predispositions, and current medications. For instance, elderly patients, with their often-diminished renal and hepatic function, are more susceptible to drug accumulation and toxicity. Similarly, patients with a history of allergies require careful scrutiny of medication choices.

A comprehensive medication review is crucial to this assessment. This involves scrutinizing all prescribed, over-the-counter, and herbal remedies a patient is taking, analyzing them for potential interactions or contraindications. This detailed evaluation should not be a one-time event, but an ongoing process, particularly when new medications are introduced or existing regimens are modified. Documentation of this process is paramount, providing a clear and accessible record for all healthcare professionals involved in the patient's care. This shared knowledge base promotes informed decision-making and minimizes the risk of conflicting treatments.

Beyond individual patient assessment, systematic approaches play a vital role. Hospitals and healthcare systems can implement standardized protocols for medication reconciliation, ensuring consistency and accuracy in medication information across different care settings. These protocols should encompass admission, transfer, and discharge, creating a seamless flow of information and minimizing the risk of medication errors during transitions of care. Regular audits of medication practices can further identify systemic weaknesses and drive continuous improvement in patient safety.

Monitoring drug therapy is the next critical step. It's akin to keeping a watchful eye on a complex chemical reaction, ready to intervene if things go awry. Regular laboratory monitoring, especially for drugs with a narrow therapeutic index, allows healthcare professionals to track drug levels and adjust dosages as needed. This proactive approach can prevent adverse events by maintaining drug concentrations within the therapeutic range, avoiding both subtherapeutic levels and toxic overexposure. Think of it as maintaining the delicate balance required for optimal therapeutic effect without undue harm.

Patient education and engagement are integral components of effective monitoring. Empowering patients with knowledge about their medications, potential side effects, and warning signs empowers them to actively participate in their own safety. Clear and concise communication, tailored to the patient's understanding, is crucial. Encourage patients to report any unusual symptoms or concerns promptly, fostering a collaborative relationship between patient and healthcare provider. This partnership creates a safety net, catching potential problems early and minimizing their impact.

Prevention strategies offer yet another layer of protection. These strategies focus on minimizing the opportunity for errors to occur in the first place. Standardized drug administration protocols, particularly in high-risk settings like intensive care units, help reduce medication errors. Implementing electronic prescribing systems can minimize errors related to illegible handwriting or misinterpretation of drug names. Furthermore, these systems can integrate alerts for potential drug interactions or contraindications, providing realtime safeguards against prescribing errors.

Effective communication among healthcare professionals is the linchpin of patient safety. A fragmented healthcare system, with information siloed in different departments or institutions, poses significant risks. Clear and concise communication channels, facilitated by electronic health records and shared databases, are essential for seamless information exchange. This collaborative environment fosters a culture of safety, where healthcare professionals share responsibility for preventing medication-related harm. Regular interdisciplinary reviews of medication practices further strengthen communication and promote continuous learning and improvement.

Consider the case of a patient prescribed a new medication. A pharmacist, reviewing the patient's medication list, identifies a potential interaction with an existing drug. By promptly communicating this concern to the prescribing physician, a potentially harmful interaction is averted. This exemplifies the power of collaborative communication in preventing adverse events. Patient safety is not the sole responsibility of any single healthcare professional but a shared commitment that requires vigilance, communication, and a proactive approach to risk management. Every interaction, every prescription, every monitoring check presents an opportunity to strengthen the safety net and protect patients from potential harm. This commitment is a continuous journey, one that demands constant learning, adaptation, and a steadfast dedication to prioritizing patient well-being.

7.1 Risk Assessment

Identifying potential drug-related risks is a critical component of patient safety. A thorough risk assessment involves a systematic evaluation of various factors that can predispose a patient to adverse drug reactions (ADRs) or negative drug interactions. This process requires a comprehensive understanding of the patient's medical history, current medications, lifestyle, and genetic predispositions. By carefully considering these individual factors, healthcare professionals can tailor medication regimens to minimize potential harm and optimize therapeutic outcomes. Effective risk assessment, therefore, serves as a cornerstone of preventative medicine, allowing for proactive intervention to safeguard patient well-being.

Risk assessment should not be viewed as a static event but rather a dynamic process. It begins with obtaining a detailed medication history. This includes not only prescription drugs but also over-the-counter medications, herbal supplements, and vitamins. Understanding the complete picture of a patient's medication intake is crucial for identifying potential interactions. For instance, a patient taking St. John's Wort, a herbal supplement, alongside certain antidepressants can experience serotonin syndrome, a potentially life-threatening condition. Therefore, eliciting a comprehensive medication history, including seemingly innocuous substances, is paramount.

Beyond medication history, a patient's medical history plays a significant role in risk assessment. Pre-existing conditions such as liver or kidney disease can significantly impact drug metabolism and excretion. For example, patients with impaired renal function are at increased risk of drug accumulation and toxicity. Similarly, liver disease can alter drug metabolism, leading to unpredictable drug levels and potentially increased ADRs. Therefore, a careful review of a patient's medical history, including laboratory results indicative of organ function, is essential for identifying potential vulnerabilities to drug-related complications.

Genetic factors also contribute significantly to individual variability in drug response. Pharmacogenomics, the study of how genes affect a person's response to drugs, offers valuable insights into potential ADR risks. Certain genetic variations can influence drug metabolism, transport, and target receptor sensitivity. For example, variations in the CYP2D6 gene can affect the metabolism of numerous medications, including certain antidepressants and antipsychotics. Knowing a patient's pharmacogenomic profile can allow for personalized medication selection and dosage adjustments, thereby mitigating the risk of ADRs. While routine pharmacogenomic testing is not yet standard practice, its increasing availability holds promise for more precise and safer drug therapy in the future.

Lifestyle factors, often overlooked, can significantly impact drug safety. Smoking, alcohol consumption, and dietary habits can interact with medications in complex ways. For instance, smoking induces certain drug-metabolizing enzymes, leading to decreased drug levels and potentially reduced efficacy. Alcohol can potentiate the sedative effects of certain medications, increasing the risk of falls and other accidents. Similarly, certain foods can interact with drugs, either enhancing or inhibiting their absorption. Therefore, inquiring about a patient's lifestyle habits is an integral part of a comprehensive risk assessment.

Age is a critical factor to consider during risk assessment. Both very young and elderly patients are at increased risk of ADRs. Infants and children have immature organ systems, leading to differences in drug absorption, distribution, metabolism, and excretion compared to adults. Elderly patients, on the other hand, often experience age-related decline in organ function, making them more susceptible to drug accumulation and toxicity. Additionally, polypharmacy, the concurrent use of multiple medications, is common in older adults, further increasing the risk of drug interactions and ADRs. Therefore, age-specific considerations are essential for ensuring safe and effective drug therapy across the lifespan.

Pregnancy and breastfeeding present unique challenges in medication management. Many drugs can cross the placenta and potentially harm the developing fetus. Similarly, drugs can be excreted in breast milk, posing risks to nursing infants. Therefore, careful consideration of the risks and benefits of any medication is crucial during pregnancy and lactation. Consulting resources such as the FDA's pregnancy categories and LactMed database can provide valuable information regarding drug safety in these populations.

Beyond individual patient factors, specific drug characteristics contribute to risk assessment. Drugs with a narrow therapeutic index, meaning the difference between the effective dose and the toxic dose is small, require particularly close monitoring. Examples include warfarin, digoxin, and lithium. Even small variations in drug levels can lead to significant adverse effects. Therefore, patients taking these medications require careful dosage adjustments and regular monitoring of drug levels to ensure therapeutic efficacy while minimizing the risk of toxicity.

Drug formulation can also influence risk. Sustained-release formulations, designed to release the drug slowly over time, can pose a risk of dose dumping, a rapid release of a large amount of the drug, if the formulation is crushed or chewed. This can lead to potentially dangerous drug levels. Therefore, patient education regarding proper administration of different drug formulations is essential.

Finally, awareness of high-alert medications is paramount in risk assessment. These are medications that have a heightened risk of causing significant patient harm when used in error. Examples include insulin, opiates, and chemotherapeutic agents. Implementing specific safety protocols for these medications, such as double-checking dosages and using independent verification, can help prevent medication errors and minimize patient harm. Through a systematic and comprehensive approach to risk assessment, healthcare professionals can significantly reduce the incidence of drug-related harm and promote safer medication practices for all patients. This approach is vital for safeguarding patient health and optimizing therapeutic outcomes.

7.2 Monitoring & Prevention

Effective monitoring and prevention strategies are paramount in minimizing drug-related harm and ensuring patient safety. This involves a multi-faceted approach encompassing vigilant observation for adverse drug reactions (ADRs), proactive risk mitigation, and fostering a culture of open communication between healthcare professionals, patients, and regulatory bodies. Implementing standardized procedures, utilizing technology, and leveraging patient education are crucial components of a comprehensive safety framework. The goal is to create a proactive system that identifies potential problems before they escalate, thereby optimizing therapeutic outcomes and safeguarding patient well-being.

Continuous monitoring of patients receiving medication is the cornerstone of preventative care. This involves not just observing for the intended therapeutic effects, but also for any signs of adverse drug reactions. These reactions can range from mild, predictable side effects, such as nausea or drowsiness, to severe and life-threatening events like anaphylaxis or organ damage. Early detection of ADRs allows for prompt intervention, mitigating potential harm. The process necessitates meticulous documentation of patient medication history, including over-the-counter drugs and supplements, allergies, and pre-existing medical conditions. Regular follow-up appointments and open communication channels for patients to report any unusual symptoms are essential elements of effective monitoring. Empowering patients to actively participate in their care significantly enhances the likelihood of early ADR detection.

Risk assessment is an integral part of preventative strategies. By identifying patients at higher risk of experiencing ADRs or drug interactions, healthcare professionals can tailor treatment plans and implement preventative measures. Factors contributing to increased risk include age, polypharmacy (taking multiple medications concurrently), pre-existing medical conditions, and genetic predispositions. Several validated risk assessment tools can assist in stratifying patients based on their individual risk profiles. Utilizing these tools enables healthcare providers to make informed decisions regarding drug selection, dosage adjustments, and the need for closer monitoring. This proactive approach minimizes the potential for adverse events and optimizes the balance between therapeutic benefit and risk.

Minimizing the risk of drug interactions is another crucial aspect of patient safety. Drug interactions occur when one drug alters the effect of another, potentially leading to reduced efficacy or increased toxicity. A thorough understanding of drug interaction mechanisms, including pharmacokinetic and pharmacodynamic interactions, is essential for healthcare professionals. Pharmacokinetic interactions affect the absorption, distribution, metabolism, and excretion of drugs, while pharmacodynamic interactions occur at the site of action. By reviewing patient medication profiles and consulting comprehensive drug interaction databases, healthcare providers can identify potential interactions and take steps to prevent them. These steps might include adjusting dosages, switching to alternative medications, or closely monitoring for signs of interaction.

Effective communication is paramount in preventing medication errors and managing ADRs. Clear and concise communication between healthcare professionals, patients, and their families is vital. This includes providing patients with detailed information about their medications, including potential side effects and precautions. Encouraging patients to ask questions and actively participate in their care empowers them to be vigilant partners in preventing drug-related harm. Open communication among healthcare professionals is equally important. Sharing information about patient medication histories, allergies, and potential drug interactions ensures that everyone involved in the patient's care is aware of potential risks. Standardized procedures for prescribing, dispensing, and administering medications, coupled with robust documentation, further minimize the likelihood of errors.

Utilizing technology can significantly enhance monitoring and prevention efforts. Electronic prescribing systems reduce medication errors by providing built-in checks for drug interactions and allergies. Automated alerts can flag potential problems and prompt healthcare providers to review and adjust prescriptions as needed. Pharmacovigilance databases, which collect and analyze reports of ADRs, are invaluable tools for identifying emerging drug safety concerns. These databases enable healthcare professionals to stay abreast of the latest safety information and make informed decisions regarding medication use. Data mining techniques applied to large datasets can also reveal patterns and trends related to ADRs, further refining risk assessment and prevention strategies.

Educating patients about their medications is a key component of patient safety. Providing clear and concise information about medication purpose, dosage, administration, potential side effects, and precautions empowers patients to actively participate in their care. This also includes advising patients on the importance of reporting any unusual symptoms to their healthcare provider. Educational materials, such as medication guides and patient counseling sessions, are valuable tools for enhancing patient understanding. When patients are well-informed about their medications, they are more likely to adhere to prescribed regimens, report potential problems promptly, and contribute to a safer medication-use environment.

The role of regulatory bodies is also critical in monitoring and preventing drug-related harm. Agencies like the Food and Drug Administration (FDA) play a crucial role in ensuring drug safety by overseeing drug development, approval, and post-marketing surveillance. They collect and analyze data on ADRs, issue safety warnings, and implement regulatory actions as needed. Healthcare professionals have a responsibility to report suspected ADRs to regulatory bodies, contributing to the ongoing monitoring of drug safety. This collective effort helps to identify and address emerging drug safety concerns and protect public health.

Through comprehensive monitoring, proactive risk assessment, effective communication, leveraging technology, patient education, and robust regulatory oversight, the incidence of drug-related harm can be significantly reduced, contributing to a safer and more effective healthcare system. Continuously evaluating and refining these strategies is essential to maintain and enhance patient safety in the ever-evolving landscape of pharmaceutical care.

www.ingramcontent.com/pod-product-compliance
Lightning Source LLC
LaVergne TN
LVHW020236210926
848481LV00016B/2342